How I Survived My Husband's Brain Injury

Casey Bachus

TATE PUBLISHING
AND ENTERPRISES, LLC

How I Survived My Husband's Brain Injury

Published by Tate Publishing & Enterprises, LLC
127 E. Trade Center Terrace | Mustang, Oklahoma 73064 USA
1.888.361.9473 | www.tatepublishing.com

Tate Publishing is committed to excellence in the publishing industry. The company reflects the philosophy established by the founders, based on Psalm 68:11,
"The Lord gave the word and great was the company of those who published it."

Cover design by Lauro Talibong
Interior design by Caypeeline Casas

Published in the United States of America

ISBN: 978-1-62510-975-0
1. Biography & Autobiography / Personal Memoirs
13.03.04

Dedication

To my loving husband, Jeff.

ACKNOWLEDGMENTS

First of all, I would like to thank God. Without his presence, I never would have made it through this journey. I thank him for the strength he provided me, for his provisions, and for the many miracles that he performed.

I would also like to thank our supportive network of family and friends. Thank you to anyone who helped us in any way. Thank you to anyone who cooked a meal, walked or fed our dogs, mowed our lawn, or cleaned our house. Thank you to everyone who helped us financially, whether it was buying a plate of food at our benefit, bidding on an auction item, or just donating money to help with our bills. Thank you to those who called in favors to help with our medical bills and provided free medical care.

I want to give a special thanks to our parents. I can't imagine what it was like to watch your children go through the pain and the hurt that we did. Thank you for being strong for us and helping us persevere during such a difficult time.

Contents

PREFACE

At the age of twenty-six, my life was turned upside down when my husband, Jeff, flew off a four-wheeler and hit his head. Just like that, my husband had a traumatic brain injury. My life would never be the same again, and neither would his. Fearful, helpless, excited, angry, frustrated, happy, confused, depressed, sad, joyful, peaceful, loved, stressed, anxiousness, awed, trusting, annoyed—these are just a few of the emotions that I have experienced through my journey. Many of them were simultaneous.

When my husband's accident happened, lots of people tried to help by putting me in contact with other people that had experienced a traumatic brain injury with someone they loved. However, it seemed like those that I was put in contact with to help me cope were moms, and the person injured was their child. I do not want to downplay their suffering. I know they have a lot of anguish in a tragedy like this, and in some ways, more than a spouse, but they don't deal with the same things that spouses do. Moms see their children much differently than wives see their husbands. I just didn't feel like I had anyone that I could really talk to who understood what I was going through for the majority of my journey.

I needed to talk to another wife, someone who understood what I was going through. I didn't feel like there were many resources that would help in the way that I was looking for. There were tons of materials out there about brain injuries, what to expect, and even from the point of view of the person that is injured, but nothing to help me cope with the emotions I was feeling. There was nothing to help me know whether what I was feeling was normal and what to do about it. I wanted to know how someone else got through their difficult circumstance. So I wrote this book specifically for other spouses from the point of view of a spouse of someone with a traumatic brain injury. However, I also want to reach out to anyone who is going through a tragedy in their life. This book is about my journey through a tragedy in mine and my husband's lives and how I got through it.

I have included many of the blogs that were written on a website we set up to keep our friends and family informed. Unless otherwise noted, they were written by me. Some notes from our guest book from the same website have also been included. I revealed many personal struggles that I had throughout this journey in hopes that it will somehow help someone else going through a difficult time. I want for anyone reading this to understand that the emotions you are struggling with are normal and that you are not the only one that has experienced this. You are not alone.

INTRODUCTION

On June 25th, around 12:30 Saturday morning, I was sitting on the steps of the back porch with Tess and Brittany watching the guys play washers. We had finished eating the delicious barbeque Jeff made and were enjoying each other's company.

Jeff and Brian stopped playing washers to start putting things away. Jeff asked Brian to help him put up the four-wheelers before Brian left. Walking there, Jeff remembered a road that he loves to drive down. He called it the Ingram Road. He wanted to show Brian.

"Come on. Let's go check it out. We'll be back before the girls even know we're gone," urged Jeff. Brian agreed, and they jumped on the four-wheelers for one last joyride before heading home.

Everything was fine. They were enjoying a leisurely ride down the winding road. Brian was behind Jeff, so he turned his head to make sure Brian was still there before heading around the next corner. Unexpectedly, the handle wouldn't turn to go around the corner, so he jerked it harder. When he did, Jeff lost control of the four-wheeler and went off the road. There was a steep incline and ditch that the vehicle got stuck in, causing Jeff to fly off it and smash his head on a tree.

He lay crumpled and bloody in the ditch next to the tree. Brian looked around, hoping to see a car coming down the road to help, but it was late, and few cars went down that road even during the day. There was no sign of help coming. He ran down to discover the severity of the situation. Jeff was breathing, but he wasn't conscious. Brian checked his pockets for his phone; it was not there. They left both their phones back at the house. He thought about driving back for help, but he didn't know if he could find his way back to Jeff. Plus, they were in the country, and there was no telling what animals might find Jeff lying there helplessly.

His only choice was to pick him up, lay Jeff across his lap, and slowly make the agonizing journey back to the house. What should have been a 5 minute ride back to the house took over 30 minutes as Brian had to stop every few minutes to adjust the limp body lying across his lap.

Little did I know, but my own agonizing journey was about to begin.

How We Met

It was the summer of 2006. I had just graduated with a BA in psychology from the University of Texas at San Antonio. I was living with my dad while I worked at my church in New Braunfels as an intern. In the fall, I planned to move to Fort Worth to get an MA in marriage and family counseling at Southwestern Baptist Theological Seminary. Leading up to this point, I had dated a lot of guys and was always looking to settle down with someone and get married.

That plan hadn't worked out so well for me. At this point in my life, I was finally content with where I was. I didn't need a man in my life and wasn't really looking for a husband anymore. I was in a transition period and just wanted to enjoy life.

My Aunt Sheila had been trying to set me up on a blind date for a while, but I had never been on one and really didn't have a desire to go on one. But she just kept bugging me about it, so I agreed just to get her off my back. I determined that if the date didn't go well, then I could hold that over her head and never have to go on another blind date again. If it went well though, I reasoned that I would have someone fun to hang out with for a couple of months until I moved. I was not looking for anything serious.

Jeff and I went on our first date on July 2, 2006. It was nothing special. We went to the bowling alley in New Braunfels. I could tell right away that there was something different about him. At six feet tall, he was taller than me, which is hard to find since I'm five-foot-nine myself. He had short, dark hair and piercing blue eyes. He was thin, weighing in at a measly 155 pounds, but he wasn't a weakling. I could see his muscles poking out when he flexed to throw the bowling ball down the lane.

While he was very good-looking, that wasn't what attracted me to him. I could tell right away that he didn't take life too seriously and loved to have fun. He was energetic and always seemed to have a smile on his face. And I loved his one-of-a-kind laugh! I could hear him in the next room and know it was him laughing. It always put a smile on my face to hear that laugh. I did tend to take life too seriously, but I had a few wild hairs on my head and enjoyed a little excitement.

We didn't just bowl a regular game; we had fun with it. I came up with the idea to spin ourselves around in a chair a few times before trying to roll the ball down the lane. He looked at me like I might be crazy but agreed to it. We had a blast, trying not to fall over before we let the ball sail down the lane toward the pins.

Afterward, I had already scheduled to go see a movie with one of my girlfriends. I wanted an excuse to leave in case the date didn't go well. It went great though, and he ended up joining us to see a chick flick on our first date. Not only was he man enough to go see this movie, he also paid for both me and my friend to get in as well. We parted ways that night and agreed to see each other again but didn't set up another date.

I don't know what I was thinking, but the following weekend, my friend was getting married, and I didn't have a date to the wedding. I didn't really want to go alone, so I invited Jeff to come with me. He agreed to go. After the wedding, some friends were going out to a ranch that someone's grandparents owned. We joined them and hung out while we danced and listened to music all night long. I couldn't pinpoint it, but there was something about him that was just different from other guys that I had dated.

My Aunt Sheila and Jeff share the same birthday, July 11. Sheila was having a birthday party at her house, so I thought it only natural to invite Jeff since she had set us up. So by our third date, he had already met most of my friends and family.

At the party, people were asking us how serious things were. I mean, who invites a guy they just met to a family member's birthday party? I explained that it was only our third date, and we weren't looking for anything serious. In the back of my mind though, I knew that there were feelings growing already. I just had this feeling that he was the one. But I wasn't looking for a boyfriend, so I pushed those thoughts out of my mind. I just wanted to have someone to do stuff with until I left.

After a few more dates, I could feel there was something between us. Driving through a park we had the awkward "define the relationship" talk. We agreed that we would be exclusive. However, I made it clear that I was moving soon, and long-distance relationships never worked out for me. We agreed to just see where this took us.

Jeff has always been very much an extrovert. I have never met anyone that didn't just love him. He has this way about him and was always very comfortable around other people. Laughter surrounded him; everyone always comments about that unique laugh of his. With me though, he seemed somewhat timid.

It took him probably five or six dates before he ever attempted to hold my hand. I remember it so vividly. We were at the movie theater, and I had my arm on the armrest between us with my hand hanging over the edge. He put his arm on it next to mine, so they were touching, and the edge of my hand was touching his. Then very slowly, as if he didn't want me to notice, he put his pinky over mine. Once he was confident that I wasn't going to pull it away, he moved his hand over, so he was holding my ring finger. He kept moving his hand over, finger by finger, until we were finally holding hands. It even took Jeff ten dates before he finally kissed me for the first time!

About two days before I was moving, we had gone on another date. The whole time, it felt like he wanted to tell me something but just couldn't get the courage to do it. I knew he wanted to tell me that he loved me, but I wasn't going to say it first. He lived in San Antonio, so on most of our dates we met halfway, and then I would get in his car to go to our destination. This night, the date was almost over, and we were standing at my car, saying goodbye. The conversation felt so awkward.

"So…did you enjoy the movie?" Jeff asked trying to stall.

"Yeah, it was good," I answered as I stared into his eyes, daring him to say those words first.

"Well, I'm not ready for you to leave yet. You want to go inside and get some hot chocolate or something?" he asked with hope in his voice. I agreed, realizing he still needed more time.

We went inside and ordered some hot cocoa. As I was taking a sip, he finally blurted out "I love you."

I laughed as I set my cup down and answered, "Well, it's about time! I love you too!"

I moved to Fort Worth and went back almost every weekend to see Jeff. He proposed after only five months. He found a job in Fort Worth, and we were married eleven months to the day that we met.

The first time that we lived in the same town, not to mention the same house, was when he moved to Fort Worth after we got married. So needless to say, we had a lot of adjustments to make. Our marriage wasn't perfect, but we worked through our problems like most married couples do. The next four years were full of challenges, but we got through them. I graduated, and we moved to New Braunfels and built a house.

I decided not to become a counselor and went into sales instead. Then I got my teaching certification and began teaching. Jeff was offered a promotion to stay in Fort Worth when he put in his two-week notice to move back to New Braunfels, so we had a long-distance marriage for a year until they relocated him to Austin.

Then after all that time waiting, he was laid off from his job. He was unemployed for six months before finding a job in New Braunfels. I guess God knew what he was doing because after living apart and commuting for a year, we were finally living and working in the same town. Our lives were right on schedule and going, for the most part, according to our plan.

Just Another Day

Friday, June 24, 2011, started out like any normal day would. As a teacher, I was enjoying the summer off. My mom, Sharon, and stepdad, James, left for Canada that morning to attend my cousin's wedding. Jeff and I were watching their dog, Holly, for the week in exchange for letting us stay at their house for the weekend. They had recently finished building their dream home complete with a courtyard, workout room, and movie room. They also had exciting toys for grown-ups such as a golf cart, four-wheelers, and Jeff's favorite, an outdoor cooking area with a built-in grill. We liked to tease them that we were going to sell our house and move in with them.

Jeff and I don't have any children, but we have two dogs that we treat as if they were our children. We have had both of them since they were puppies and before we were married. We call each other's dog our stepchild. Jeff's dog is a Great Dane, and he named her Chicken. I have a little twenty-pound mutt named Buddie.

I woke up that morning and took our dogs to my parents'. We (the dogs and I) had a leisurely day of running on the treadmill, lying out in the courtyard to work on my tan, and watching movies on the big screen HD TV. Jeff was at his new job where he worked in the IT department. He loved it, and everyone there seemed to love having him.

That evening, we planned to have some friends over for a barbecue and to play with some of the toys at the house. Jeff is a fun-loving guy and enjoyed hanging out with people. The new grill at my parents' house was the perfect excuse to have a barbecue. The evening was going just as planned. We took the four-wheelers out for a ride as well as the golf cart. Jeff cooked some delicious fajitas.

Later in the night, the people left were our neighbors Tess, Brian, and Brittany. The guys were playing washers in the backyard while I sat with Tess and Brittany on the steps, watching them. We were talking about how blessed we felt. I was sharing with them about how blessed I was to be married to a man as wonderful as Jeff and how great our marriage was.

It seemed that in the past few weeks, we had felt closer than ever. While we may not have had a life that the world would be jealous of, we were living an abundant life. We had faith in God, and he was blessing us. We enjoyed the time we had together and were thankful for what we had been blessed with. It was nice to enjoy some of the added luxuries that my parents had, but we were relishing in the life that we had been blessed with.

I had just come out of a valley spiritually. I went through a few years where I was not seeking God. I wasn't blatantly disobeying him, but I wasn't following him. Most people probably didn't even notice a difference. I had been a Christian long enough that I knew how to talk the talk. However, in 2010 and 2011, I was getting back on track again. I was seeking God again, and my relationship with him was growing.

Jeff and I had just celebrated our four-year anniversary. We made it through a few challenges and had come out victorious on the other side. We both had good jobs. We built our first house and had been living in it for almost two years. Jeff and I were beginning to discuss the option of starting a family together. We knew we wanted to wait awhile longer but were talking about starting our family in the next couple years. We were happy and enjoying the life we had together. Little did I know that my world was about to be turned completely upside-down. The picture-perfect life we were living was about to be shattered to pieces.

The Accident

I was sitting on the steps of the back porch with Brittany and Tess. We were watching the guys play washers while we talked about life. The guys left to put the four wheelers up, and we continued talking. It was great enjoying some girl time and sharing how our lives were going at the moment. We were all lighthearted and having a great time. Then we realized the guys hadn't come back yet.

"How long has it been since the guys left to put the four-wheelers up?" I asked.

"I'm not sure, it's been a while though. Surely it wouldn't take this long. I have a feeling something is wrong." Tess answered.

"I'm sure everything is fine," I stated, knowing Jeff is a fun-loving guy. I assumed they were just out taking a joyride.

We hopped in the golf cart and went searching for them. We got down to the end of the street, and the battery started to die. "We better turn around before we get stuck out there. Let's go back and get the car," I told them.

We went back to the house and got in Brittany's car. "Something is wrong, I have this feeling," Tess insisted.

"Nothing is wrong, Tess. They are just out goofing around. You know those guys. I bet Jeff took Brian to see the Ingram Road," I assured her.

We started driving back out of the driveway. Right about that time, we saw one pair of headlights from a four-wheeler coming up the driveway.

"There they are. See, I told you they were fine!" I exclaimed. Then we realized that the second pair of headlights didn't follow. That's when my heart sank.

"Why is there only one set of headlights?" Tess asked with fear in her voice.

Still not wanting to accept anything bad had happened, I reasoned, "I bet the battery died on the other one. That's what took them so long."

Then as they got closer, I realized that Brian was carrying Jeff's unconscious body on his four-wheeler.

I was in the backseat of Brittany's two-door Camaro. When they saw the guys, both of them jumped out of the car, leaving me in the backseat. I was screaming at them to let me out, panicking and trying to push the seat up myself so I could climb out of the car. They must have been afraid to let me out because they didn't want me to see Jeff. Tess pushed the seat up though, and I leaped out of the vehicle. Jeff's limp body was lying across Brian's lap. Brian had taken his shirt off to wrap around Jeff's bloody head.

My first thought was, *This can't be happening. We don't have insurance!* When my friends said we needed to call an ambulance, I told them it didn't look that bad and we could just drive him. They looked at me like I was insane and said we had to get an ambulance. That's when it began to sink in. I made the 911 call.

"Is he conscious?" the operator asked calmly on the other end of the phone. I looked at Jeff just lying there; I looked at Tess and Brian and repeated the question to them. Only, there was no sign of calm in my voice.

"No!" I said.

Just as calmly as before, the operator asked, "Is he breathing?" I didn't know. My eyes widened as the severity of what was happening began to sink in. I started yelling the questions at Brian in terror. He assured me that Jeff was breathing. After a few minutes, Tess took the phone, and I was told to go wait by the house so I didn't have to see Jeff like that.

I began to go into shock. While we were waiting, I remember feeling very calm and organized, in a panicked kind of way. I ran back in the house and grabbed my purse and overnight bag. Since we were already packed, I figured it didn't hurt to take it. I felt silly doing it because I thought surely they would just take him to the hospital, he would be fine, and we could go home.

My heart was racing, and I had tunnel vision. I felt like I was on autopilot. I was trying to think of everything that I needed or needed to do before we left. At the same time, I wasn't thinking; I wasn't processing. My mind was blank yet full simultaneously.

When the ambulance got there, they put Jeff in a drug-induced coma to take over his breathing. I tried to show the EMS crew that I was all right by offering information. I was spouting off his birthday, social security number, medical history, anything I thought would help them. The crew told me they thought he had fractured his skull. They tried twice to airlift him to the hospital, but the helicopters weren't able to get there. I rode in the ambulance to the first hospital. The whole way, I kept muttering under my breath, "Okay, Okay, Okay, Okay," over and over. I don't know why; I guess I was just processing everything.

We got to the first hospital to wait for the second airlift attempt to a hospital in San Antonio. The helicopter got all the way there. I could see it getting ready to land; then suddenly, it turned away and left.

The EMS said they got a call for somebody worse than Jeff. They didn't want me to ride in the ambulance to San Antonio, so I got in the car with Brittany. The car ride from the hospital in New Braunfels to the one in San Antonio was the longest ride of my life. Growing up in New Braunfels, I have made the drive to San Antonio many times, but it never took as long as it did that night. Time was standing still. I had a million thoughts running through my mind; then, I would look out the window and realize we had only gone a mile or two.

I didn't know how bad it was, so I didn't know if I should call our families yet. I didn't know how to make that kind of phone call. I decided to call our parents. It was about 2:00 a.m. when I started calling. No one was answering their phones. I couldn't bring myself to leave a message, so I just kept trying. I had been trying for a few hours to get ahold of them and couldn't.

By that time, we were at the hospital, and I knew it was pretty serious. So I sent out an e-mail to our small group at church because I knew that people needed to be praying. It said, "Uh, I've been trying to get ahold of our parents first, but they aren't answering, and we need prayer. Jeff was in a bad accident and is in ICU right now. He has severe head trauma and isn't responding. I don't know much more than that, just please pray."

I eventually started calling Jeff's sisters, hoping they would answer and could go wake up his parents. One of his sisters finally answered; by that time, it was 6:00 a.m. It doesn't matter how much I practiced that call in my head, actually saying the words was another story.

When I heard the voice on the other end of the phone, I tried to stay as calm as possible. "Jeff's been in an accident."

I could hear the panic in his sister's voice. "Is he okay?"

"I don't know," was all I could choke out before I started crying. I told her I'd been trying to call his mom, but she wasn't answering. I told her where we were, and she said she would get ahold of their family and get there as soon as possible.

When I finally got to the hospital, I could barely walk; I was in so much shock. Brittany had to help me into the hospital. Every room we were moved to, I was looking for the trashcan because I felt like I was going to throw up at any moment. We waited for hours. They told us that he was stable but still unconscious. They were running tests and doing CAT scans and X-rays. A chaplain came by several times to talk and pray with us.

I was sitting in the waiting room with Brittany, Tess, and Brian. We didn't know what to do or say or how to feel. I tried to hold it together, but sometimes, I couldn't do anything but put my face in my hands and cry. However, right about the time I would start, a doctor or someone would come in the room and start talking to us, so I would try to pull myself back together.

In the midst of it, my friends tried to lighten the mood a little. Laughter helped me immensely through this journey. It helped to keep me sane. Jeff made everything into a joke, so by joking about the situation, it made me feel more connected to him. I remember Tess was wearing sandals, and her feet were black from walking in the dirt. She wanted to wash them off. There was a water fountain in the waiting room, so she stuck her foot in it to wash it off! We started cracking up. Looking back, I don't know why she didn't just go to find a restroom, but it lightened the mood a little.

At one point, it was just Brittany and I in the waiting room. There was a lot of sitting in silence. There were so many thoughts running through my mind. It helped to have someone sitting next to me. I finally understood the verses in Job when his friends arrived. "Then they sat on the ground with him for seven days and seven nights. No one said a word to him, because they saw how great his suffering was" (Job 2:13). I always struggled with what to do or say when someone is hurting the way I was. I learned that night that sometimes the best thing to do is sit quietly next to them while they work through all the torments in their head.

They finally let me see him around 4:30 a.m. I had talked Brian and Tess into leaving to take care of their children, and I still hadn't been able to get ahold of our family, so Brittany was the only one there with me. We walked into the room, and she had her arm around my shoulder. I don't know what I expected when I walked in there, but it wasn't what I saw.

There was my husband, lying on a hospital bed. He looked lifeless. There were tubes everywhere. A massive tube was shoved into his throat connected to a machine that breathed for him. It caused his chest to rise and fall mechanically. He had wires attached to his chest, arms, and hands. There was a cervical collar around his neck, holding his head in place. There was a giant gash on the right side of his head where he hit the tree, and blood was oozing from it. He had scratches on his arms and legs. A hospital gown covered the rest of his body.

I wanted to crawl in the bed and hold him. I wanted to wrap my arms around him and tell him that everything was going to be all right, that I loved him, and that I wasn't angry that he had left without telling me. I looked at one of the nurses standing next to me and asked if I could get in the bed with him. She looked back at me alarmed and told me no. It must have sounded like a crazy question, but I just wanted to hold him. Instead, I held his hand and, between sobs, began telling him how much I love him.

We only had a few minutes. Right before I came in the room, I was told that he had stopped responding again, and he would have to be rushed back to do another CAT scan. He had three bleeds in his brain, and they wanted to make sure they weren't worsening.

We sat for a couple more hours in the waiting room, and our immediate family started trickling in. The results of the second CAT scan finally came back, and it revealed that there were no new bleeds in Jeff's brain, and he had started responding to pain again. We were allowed to start going in to see him two at a time. He was hooked up to all kinds of machines. He wasn't breathing on his own and was still unconscious.

It was explained that Jeff wasn't in a coma, but he was unconscious; although, there wasn't much difference. Had he stayed in that state for much longer, they would have classified it as a coma. The only thing he responded to was pain, and then it was just a general moving or squirming to ease the pain. It was not purposeful movement. He didn't open his eyes or try to move the object away that was causing pain. The doctors had to induce pain every hour to make sure that he still responded. If he stopped, it was a sign that he was getting worse.

Waiting for Answers

The first twenty-four to forty-eight hours are supposed to be the most critical. If Jeff didn't wake up in that time frame, then we knew that he was worse than what was expected. If he didn't wake up before the forty-eight-hour mark, I was told not to expect him to wake up shortly after that. It could take days, weeks, months, or possibly not ever. I wanted him to wake up now, but especially before the forty-eight hours were up. Time was flying by and standing still at the same time. The forty-eight-hour window was ticking by; I hadn't slept, and the days began to run together. Yet every minute that passed that Jeff didn't wake up felt like a day.

Not a lot happened in the first twenty-four hours. There was a lot of crying on my part, but I wanted to hold it together for everyone else, so I did a lot of my crying when I was in the room alone with Jeff. I don't know why, but I felt like I had to be strong for everyone else. I felt like everyone was looking to me for direction. I was afraid that if I lost control of my emotions in front of Jeff's family, then they would lose it, too. On the other hand, I was afraid that if I didn't break down in front of them, they were going to think that I didn't love him.

I didn't know what to do, so I kept it together as much as I could in front of everyone else. I didn't even want to break down in front of my family because I knew that knowing how much I really hurt would hurt them, and I didn't want anyone else to hurt more than they already were.

In the waiting room, there were so many blank stares and faces that were void of hope and streaked with tears. Everyone looked beaten down and empty. I could see the faces of Jeff's parents and sisters. I knew I needed to try to console them, but I didn't know what to do about it. I was too grief stricken myself to worry about trying to help anyone else get through this. The only thing I felt I was able to do for anyone else was appear strong. I was the one that everyone was looking to. If I held it together, maybe it would help them.

I was reminded of the poem "Footprints in the Sand" by Mary Stevenson during this time.

> One night I had a dream
> I dreamed I was walking along the beach with the Lord
> and across the sky flashed scenes from my life.
> For each scene I noticed two sets of footprints,
> one belonged to me and the other to the Lord.
>
> When the last scene of my life flashed before me,
> I looked back at the footprints in the sand.
> I noticed that many times along the path of my life,
> there was only one set of footprints.
> I also noticed that it happened
> at the very lowest and saddest times in my life.
>
> This really bothered me
> and I questioned the Lord about it.
> "Lord, you said that once I decided to follow you,
> you would walk with me all the way,
> but I have noticed that during the most troublesome times
> in my life there is only one set of footprints.
> I don't understand why in times when I needed you most,
> you should leave me."
>
> The Lord replied, "My precious, precious child,
> I love you and I would never, never leave you

during your times of trial and suffering. "
When you saw only one set of footprints,
it was then that I carried you."

I put a picture of footprints in the sand on my phone screensaver to remind me of that poem. God carried me through the darkest time in my life. People kept telling me that I was strong, and they didn't know how I was coping with everything so well. It's because I wasn't doing anything; God was carrying me. I never would have made it through this journey without him. It was only through God's strength that I was able to endure this hardship in my life.

When people would tell me that I was strong, I thought, *What other choice do I have? Fall apart? Cry uncontrollably? Be a miserable wreck and not be able to do anything else?* I felt like I didn't have a choice but to do what I was doing. I was surviving. I was living day-by-day, hour-by-hour, minute-by-minute. I did what I had to in order to make sure my husband was getting the care that he needed. I had to keep it together so I could understand what the doctors were telling me and then go and tell everyone else.

"I love you, Lord, my strength. The Lord is my rock, my fortress and my deliverer; my God is my rock, in whom I take refuge, my shield and the horn of my salvation, my stronghold" (Psalm 18:1–2). God had taken me to a place where my only choice was to rely on him and his strength. Without it, I never would have survived. I would have become an emotional wreck, gone into a dark place in my mind, and may never have found my way out.

By Saturday morning, people were flooding in to support us. Word was spreading like a wildfire. My phone was inundated with texts, calls, and e-mails from people that wanted me to know they cared. Friends and family came in from out of town to support us. Pastors from our church came. Pastors from my dad's church came. Friends from our small group at church came. My family was there; his family was there, not just immediate family, but cousins, aunts, uncles, even distant relatives we hadn't talked to in a while. It was amazing to see the support and know that we were loved.

My mom and stepdad had gone to Canada for my cousin's wedding. They had just left that Friday morning. They weren't supposed to return until the following weekend. I agonized over whether to call them. I felt so bad calling and ruining their vacation. I rationalized that they couldn't do anything from there, and I didn't want them to have to fly back early. I just couldn't bring myself to make another phone call like that. My dad finally had to call them for me. They couldn't get a flight out until Sunday, but they took the earliest one they could get.

I was unable to sleep at all. I had been up since Friday morning, but sleep just wasn't coming. All day Saturday I was encouraged to take a nap, but I couldn't leave Jeff, and the waiting room was too noisy. Finally, in the afternoon, the nurses cleared out Jeff's room of all the visitors and told me to lie down in the recliner in the room to sleep. I tried. I lay there for almost an hour, but sleep eluded me. Worry clouded my mind. How could I sleep when Jeff was lying in that hospital bed, and we didn't know if he was going to live or die?

Despite the constant urgings from everyone, I was unwilling to go any further away from Jeff than the waiting room. I could not even bring myself to go downstairs to the food court until Sunday. I feared that the moment I left, Jeff would take a turn for the worse. I couldn't be away from him. I had to be there in case he needed me. What I could do, I didn't know, but I felt it was necessary to be close to Jeff. I was encouraged to eat, but my stomach was in knots. Someone brought me a bagel, but I was only able to eat half of it. Nothing seemed to have any flavor to it. I knew I needed to keep my strength up, but I couldn't make myself eat. Nevertheless, I am usually a stress eater, and when someone brought a bag of snickers to the waiting room, I indulged in a few—and by a few, I mean the whole bag.

That night, Saturday, I stayed at the hospital again. But this time, I was surrounded by family. My Aunt Sheila, Jeff's mom, one of his sisters, and two of his aunts, who had come in from out of town, all stayed the night with me. We took over one of the waiting rooms and lay on the couches. My aunt gave me something to help me sleep, and after thirty-six hours of running on pure adrenaline, I finally slept for a few hours.

Struggling with God

I grew up in a Christian home. My parents were both Christians, and I was taught to go to church every Sunday. I knew about God. I knew about Christ. I knew right from wrong. The knowledge was all there, it was the *relationship* with Christ that was lacking. For the most part, I was a good kid. In class, I was the teacher's pet. I was a people pleaser, until I hit high school.

About halfway through my freshman year, I met a boy. He showed me that there was this whole life out there that my parents were keeping from me. I got tired of being the good girl all the time, and I rebelled from everything my parents taught me. For about a year, I did everything I was told not to do. I had to learn my mistakes the hard way, and I did. I wasn't sure what I believed about God anymore. That was what my parents believed in, and like most teenagers, I didn't think my parents were right about anything at that stage of my life. I began researching all types of different religions. I was fascinated by spirituality, contacting the dead and even witchcraft. I didn't know what the truth was, so I began creating my own religion. Pieces were taken from the different religions that I learned about, and my own truths emerged.

Then some friends of mine started inviting me to a youth group at another church. I started going, but it was mostly to hang out with them. I thought maybe I might meet some cute guys. On New Year's Eve of 2000, I went to an overnight retreat with that youth group. I went because a guy that I liked was going, and it was an excuse to spend some time with him.

Something unexpected happened though. After all the fun and games, and right before the countdown to the New Year, there was a speaker. I don't remember what he talked about that night, but I do remember that he asked if anyone had made some mistakes and was ready to give their life to Jesus and start new, to come down to the front. So I did. I went and talked with someone and prayed a prayer to ask Jesus into my heart. I remember thinking it was a little weird because I already knew who Jesus was, and I didn't really understand what they wanted me to do, but I did it anyway. Something changed in me that night even though I didn't know what it was.

I kept going to the youth group, but instead of going to hang out, I started listening to the messages. I began to learn about having a relationship with Jesus instead of just knowing who he was. That February, I accepted another invitation to commit my life to Jesus. I prayed the prayer again. Only, the second time, I understood what it was that I was praying. After that, I began to purposefully make changes to my life. I had a relationship with Jesus, and I grasped what that meant. My life had to change because I was grateful for what Christ had done for me, and I wanted to live my life for him instead of for myself.

That doesn't mean I became this perfect girl who never made any more mistakes. I made plenty of them; I still do. I traveled through many mountains and valleys with God. Sometimes I was on fire and couldn't get enough of God. Other times, I ran from him and made really bad decisions. There were times when I was somewhere in between those two extremes, too. Just because I had given my life to Christ, didn't mean that I was immune from making mistakes. However, no matter how far I ran from God, I was his child; I had committed my life to serve him, and he always brought me back to himself.

I had been in a good place in my relationship with God leading up to the accident, but I quickly learned that it's easy to talk about prayer and how to pray when you've never been through something traumatic. It's easy to tell someone what they are supposed to do or pray in a time like this. It's something else completely when you are in the midst of tragedy.

Pastors that we knew were constantly in and out of the hospital. They would come in and pray over Jeff. Then some of them would go out in the waiting room and pray with our family. I was so grateful for that because I was too hurt and too in shock to pray. The only prayer that I could muster up those first couple days was "God, please. God, please." I didn't even know what I was asking. Those were the only two words I could get out.

I was sitting next to Jeff's bed. It was just him and me in the room. I looked at him, wanting to pray but not knowing what to say. Was I supposed to pray for him to wake up so he could be a vegetable for the rest of his life? Was I supposed to pray that he would die so he didn't have to endure whatever lay ahead? Was I supposed to pray for a miracle? I had no idea what or how to pray. So I just held Jeff's hand and said over and over, "God, please!"

I remember telling my best friend that I felt bad that I couldn't pray. I wanted to; I wasn't angry with God and not talking to him. I just didn't know what or how to pray at that moment. She told me that the Holy Spirit was interceding for me, and he knew my needs more than I did.

> In the same way, the Spirit helps us in our weakness. We do not know what we ought to pray for, but the Spirit himself intercedes for us through wordless groans. And he who searches our hearts knows the mind of the Spirit, because the Spirit intercedes for God's people in accordance with the will of God (Romans 8:26–27).

That provided some peace in my mind about the situation. I was trusting in God to get me through this; I just couldn't talk to him. It helped to know that I didn't need to. God knew my heart's desires. He could hear through my sobs and knew what I needed even before I did.

My faith in God is very strong. I trust him. Even in a tragedy like this, I knew that he would provide. Still, trusting God and living out the reality of what he was wanting me to trust him in were two very different things. I knew that he would get me through this, but that didn't mean that I wanted to go through it.

My mind was so full of emotions, thoughts, and questions that I wasn't able to do much except sit. I tried to read a couple times but found myself having to read the same paragraph five times because I couldn't focus on anything. I wasn't reading the Bible for the same reason. Jeff and I had started reading through it together before his accident, and I thought it would be good to continue doing that. Even though I wasn't able to read on my own, I was able to read out loud to Jeff. I started reading in Matthew and read about all the miracles that Jesus performed. I wanted him to perform one of those miracles on Jeff.

While I knew that God was in control and he was going to take care of everything, I was scared out of my mind. I truly struggled through this time. I never doubted God, but I just felt inadequate. At this point in the journey, I didn't care what God's will was for our lives. I was in pain. I didn't care what greater plan God had in store. All I cared about was God healing my husband and going back to the way things were before.

A few days after the accident, I sat in the bathtub, just bawling my eyes out and screaming at God. I told him that I knew I was supposed to pray for his will and that I knew he must have some great plans, but I didn't care. I didn't want to walk down the road on which he was about to take me. I wanted him to fix things. I wanted my husband back. I was pouring out my raw emotions to God. I wasn't worried about hurting his feelings; I knew he understood my hurt and pain and was big enough to take anything I said. I wanted to make sure he knew the agony that he was allowing me to endure, and I wanted him to take it away.

I usually tried to pray for God's will, but I just couldn't. I was in too much pain to care. I felt like that kind of prayer wasn't what I was supposed to be praying, so I didn't pray very often. I felt so insufficient. I felt like such a hypocrite. I thought that I should be on my knees in prayer all the time, and I just couldn't. I couldn't talk to God except to tell him that he needed to fix my husband.

And I was still so confused about how to pray. I struggled with praying for God's will versus praying for what I wanted to happen. I knew the verse, "Ask and it will be given to you, seek and you will find, knock and the door will be opened to you" (Matthew 7:7). I knew that if my will was in line with God's will, then he would grant any prayer request I asked. But I also knew, "When you ask you do not receive, because you ask with wrong motives, that you may spend what you get on your pleasures" (James 4:3). If my will wasn't in line with his, would he still grant it? I had prayed for things selfishly before; those didn't always turn out the way that I had hoped or thought they would. I didn't want to pray for something because it would make things easier in the moment, but worse in the long run. So, was I supposed to pray for a miracle, or was I supposed to pray that God's will be done?

Thankfully, that stage didn't last long. God helped me through it all, and he helped me to trust him even in the midst of great tragedy. He helped me learn how to really rely on him, and eventually he taught me how to pray. He showed me that he is greater and more powerful than anything else and that he was in control, not the doctors, not the nurses, not the statistics, not me and my stubbornness, but God, and only God.

Settling In

Under normal circumstances, people would describe me as put-together or professional. I usually take pride in my appearance. Whenever I left the house, I made sure that my hair was fixed, my makeup was on, and my clothes looked nice.

This, however, was not a normal circumstance. Vanity had been thrown out the window along with my hopes and dreams for the future. My long, dark-brown hair was pulled back in a greasy ponytail because I had not been home to take a shower in three days. I was concerned about comfort, not fashion. For the next two months, my attire consisted of T-shirts, sports bras, and workout pants. I wore my glasses because my brown eyes were too sore from crying to wear my contacts. It was futile to attempt wearing makeup because it would just run down my face or be wiped away with my tears.

I learned that what I thought was important, in the reality of the life I was living now, meant nothing. The things that I worried about before faded away in the face of the worries that lay ahead. Asking, "How do I look?" didn't matter when I was asking, "Will he live?" or "Will he remember me when he wakes up?"

In her book *The God Who Sees You*, Tammy Maltby compares trauma to living in a war zone.

> In war, everything you do is focused on survival. You are constantly in crisis, constantly running on adrenaline, slogging through rice paddies or deserts with your meager belongings in little carts or on your back, dodging bul-

> lets, crawling on your belly, doing whatever you must to survive.[1]

This is exactly how I felt. I was slogging through the hospital hallways, carrying only what was necessary for hygiene in a small bag. I was dodging the bullets of grief and despair, crawling in hopes that the worst of it would pass over me. I wasn't living; I was surviving.

The doctors were hoping that by Sunday morning, Jeff would be breathing independently on a consistent basis, and they could take him off the ventilator. However, his breathing was still sporadic. He did start opening his eyes, but it wasn't voluntary; they would only jerk open in response to pain. A feeding tube was finally inserted so he could get some nutrients, as he had not received anything since Friday night at our barbecue.

The outpouring of love during this time was amazing. I was inundated with calls, visitors, texts, and emails. It was great to know how loved we were during such a difficult time. It wasn't until Sunday night that I finally agreed to go home, while a couple of Jeff's family members stayed with him.

While Jeff was unconscious, there were so many things that happened that scared me senseless. I didn't know how I was going to live the rest of my life, let alone how Jeff was going to live his. The doctors couldn't tell me anything about what he was going to be like when/if he woke up. They were unable to answer most of my questions with anything other than, "We won't know until he wakes up." From the information that was given, the picture being painted was very dark.

For starters, Jeff hit the front, right part of his head on the tree. However, his injuries were not limited to frontal lobe damage. Jeff's injury was called a diffuse axonal injury. That means that there wasn't just one part of his brain that was affected; his entire brain was damaged. The doctors told me that his personality could change. They said that his likes and dislikes could change. Basically, when or if he woke up, he could be a completely different person from the man that I married. That terrified me.

Throughout this entire process, there were only a handful of people that saw me really break down, where I let my walls down and showed how broken I felt inside. My mom was one of those people. She stayed with me at the hospital Monday night, and I just couldn't keep it in any longer.

After my conversations with the doctors, I had fears brewing inside that I was too afraid to ask. I was afraid of what the answer might be. I needed to talk to someone, and as much as I didn't want to make her hurt even more by seeing me in so much emotional pain, I had to let it out. We had fixed up the couches in the waiting room to go to sleep, and I crawled over on the couch with my mom.

I told her that my biggest fear in all of this wasn't that Jeff would die. I knew that if he died, he was going to heaven. My biggest fear was that he was going to wake up and not like me anymore and that he would not love me.

I was petrified that his interests would change so much that he wouldn't *want* me anymore. What if I went through this torture only for Jeff to wake up and decide he didn't want to be married to me any longer? My mom just put her arms around me and let me cry and talk it out. I knew she didn't have the answers, but she tried to comfort me as best she could. I finally let myself cry a little bit that night while I was being held. It helped so much just to be in someone's arms, and knowing that no matter what happened, I had people that loved me.

Once I was finally coming to terms with my fears and was brave enough to want to know the answer, I finally asked the doctor, "If Jeff wakes up, is it possible that he won't like me anymore? Could he remember me but decide that he no longer likes who I am and doesn't want to be married to me?"

Sympathy filled his eyes. "I have never seen that happen before. It is highly unlikely that he wouldn't want you anymore. His likes and dislikes may be different, but it is usually much smaller things like his taste in food. If he liked pepperoni before, he may not like it now. It is not likely that the changes would be so major that he wouldn't like *you* anymore." I breathed a huge sigh of relief after that conversation.

However, even if Jeff still liked me, I was worried that I might not like him anymore. I wasn't going to divorce him, but would he be the same man I married? Would he still be fun loving and make me laugh? Or would he be a completely different person that I didn't know or even want to know?

That same day, another doctor came in, and I was told that Jeff might never wake up. He informed me that not only was it possible that he would never wake up, but also that I could take him home while he was still unconscious.

"I don't want to upset you, but I want to be realistic here. I want to prepare you for the worst, but you can hope for the best," he said.

It was just one extreme to the next. As soon as I felt relieved of one fear, another one surfaced. This doctor told me that he would be in a more stable condition than he was, but there was a very real possibility that I could take Jeff home while he was still unconscious. I would have to feed him through a tube, change him when he used the restroom, give him sponge baths, brush his teeth, turn him every two hours to keep him from getting bedsores, and make sure that he didn't attempt to pull his tubes out. He could live days, weeks, or even years like that.

I'm sure I was informed that if Jeff woke up, he would have a long recovery process of relearning how to walk, talk, and do all his activities of daily living, but I don't remember any of it in the first few days. In my mind, I pictured two scenarios: The first was that he would never wake up, and I would have to care for him the rest of my life. The second, I envisioned that he would wake up and not want me anymore. He would have a different personality, be a completely different person, and not want to be married to me anymore. I know the doctor reassured me the second scenario wouldn't happen, but it still weighed heavily in my mind.

While I was concerned about Jeff, I was also selfishly worried about my own future. We were young. We had only been married for four years. We didn't have children yet. I was twenty-six, and he was thirty-one. We still had our entire lives ahead of us. We had so much planned for our futures, so much more to do. And now, this was going to be my reality. This was going to be the rest of my life. Good-bye, hopes and dreams. Good-bye, future that I had imagined. Good-bye, raising a family together.

I was going to live out my vows, "For better or for worse, in sickness and in health." I was giving up every hope and dream that I had ever had for our future together. I wasn't going to get to raise children. I wasn't going to get to be the stay-at-home mom I always dreamed of being. I wasn't going to get to grow old and retire with the love of my life.

I was going to take care of my husband. I was going to raise him. I was going to have to find a way to work and take care of him. My life as I knew it was over. Yet somehow, God gave me a peace. I didn't freak out. I didn't run away screaming. I didn't even get angry with God. I just started trying to figure out how I was going to make it work. This was my new reality; now I had to figure out how to make it work.

The doctors were hoping Jeff would wake up in the first one to two days, but that didn't happen. After that, they didn't know when, or if, Jeff would wake up, and they couldn't tell me what it would be like if he did. It was impossible to predict the kind of cognitive injuries that Jeff may have suffered at this stage. All we could do was wait for him to begin awakening. Only then would they have a clearer picture of the extent of his injuries and what that would mean for us in the future.

Once they were confident that he would live, the new questions became, "What kind of life would he live?" "Would he be confined to a bed for the rest of his life?" "Was he going to be a vegetable?" "Would he ever be able to talk again?" The questions rushed through my mind like a river breaking through a dam. Nonetheless, I had to put them aside. I couldn't dwell on the "what ifs." I had to live moment by moment and take each day as it came. I couldn't think about the future because it was so uncertain.

Despite their lack of answers, some of the doctors did try to encourage me. It was explained many times that the brain is like a highway. There are neurons that fire along specific paths or highways. In Jeff's brain, many of these highways had been torn down. Now his brain was working to find and build new roads to carry the information. They explained that he had his young age and intelligence in his favor. His mind would be able to form new highways easier than someone in his same health that was older. The reconstruction in his brain would continue throughout his recovery, but they still were unable to tell me what it would look like. They just kept telling me that he was lucky this happened while he was still young.

I had to make decisions about feeding tubes and whether to leave him on the ventilator or have a tracheotomy, where they insert a breathing tube through his neck. There was a setting on the respirator that indicated if Jeff's own breaths were deep enough or close enough together, then he could breathe by himself. If they weren't, the machine would do it for him. Jeff would breathe on his own, on and off, but not consistently. I felt like if I let them perform the tracheotomy, I was accepting that he wasn't going to wake up soon. I didn't want to give up hope that he could wake up at any moment.

Jeff's family was there and wanted to be included in the decision-making. Legally, it was my decision. I didn't have to do anything they wanted. But I knew this was their son and their brother. I wanted to include them in the decisions, but ultimately, I had the final say. When he went home, he was going home with me. I had to be all right with whatever consequences would result from any decisions that were made because I would be the one that would be living with those consequences.

This is not to say that I didn't care what they had to say, or understand that they were going through the same journey, I was just in a different position. Jeff was the baby of the family and the only boy. He is his mom's pride and joy. He has always been very close to his family. His mom has continually treated me like one of her own. I never felt like a daughter-in-law with her. She tried to reach out to me in those first few days, but I didn't know how to respond. I may have been the oldest child in my family, but I was the youngest by six years in his. I was too young to be dealing with circumstances like these. I had only been part of Jeff's family for four years.

In the past when I faced difficult circumstances, I sought out wisdom from people that I knew for a long time and trusted their opinion, people that had proven their wisdom to me in the past. I had one close friend and my parents that I usually ran to. I had never leaned on his parents or sisters for wisdom before, and I didn't know their source of advice. Would their opinion be based on fear, or would they seek God's wisdom and offer advice based on prayer?

I recognized that Jeff's family had loved him a lot longer than I had. His parents brought him into this world and raised him. Without them, I wouldn't be married to this wonderful man. Ultimately, the struggles early on were mostly in my head because I generally just agreed with whatever the doctors recommended. I guess it speaks to how young and naïve I was and how ill-equipped I was to be in the middle of such a tragedy.

During this stage, I felt so many emotions all at once. I was terrified and felt so hopeless and helpless. There were moments of excitement when it looked like Jeff was making some minute progress. Through all of it though, I did have a sense of peace. I knew that no matter what happened, somehow God would get me through it. I trusted God, but, at the same time, I didn't know how to. I knew he was in control, but I was afraid of what he thought I could handle. I had a choice; I could either trust God and accept the peace he was trying to give me, or I could panic, fall apart, and go crazy because nothing was in my control. I chose to trust God.

That doesn't mean I hit my knees praying or that I ran and opened my Bible to find truth. I simply let go. I still wasn't in a place emotionally or spiritually where I could pray. I couldn't read anything even if I tried because I couldn't make my mind focus on anything except how Jeff was doing.

There have been so many things throughout this journey that I have struggled with and wondered if that struggle is normal or if it's something over which I should be stressing about. Some of them seemed so selfish. I often wondered how I could be thinking of myself in a time like this. But the reality was that if I didn't take care of myself, I wouldn't be able to take care of Jeff. I also came to realize that applied to more than just eating right and getting enough sleep. That was true for my emotional well-being also.

SLEEPOVERS

For at least the first week or two, when I did go home, I didn't want to be alone. My friends and family took turns spending the night at my house to keep me company. The first night I went home, my cousin Elise stayed with me. Elise was thirteen years old at the time, and we've always been really close. I used to babysit her a lot when she was a baby, and we would spend weeks together in the summer. I asked her to write about her experience that night.

> Accident. A small word that can mean big things. Such as a baby knocking over a bottle or even spilling something on the floor, but it can also mean a crash. In our case the "accident" was a crash.
>
> My cousin Jeff was in an accident on June 25, 2011. I found out while I was in Boston, Massachusetts. Because I was too far away to do anything, all I could do was worry. Luckily we were already planned to leave that day so I took the plane home. My cousins picked my mom, my stepdad, and I up from the airport. On the way to the hospital they tried to update us on the situation. Everything they were saying was way over my head, and the only parts I could pick out were not good. We arrived at the hospital and the mood of the family wasn't in the least bit happy. Everyone was staring off into space, thinking, wondering, praying. I felt the tension in the room and wanted to do the only thing I knew how, try to make people happier.

I brought some smiles to people's faces but they shortly went back to blankness.

I wasn't able to see Jeff, however, I did see Casey. She was being unbelievably strong in the time where we all expected her to be the opposite. She was being like superman although not even kryptonite was slowing her down.

I had to go home later that night, but my mom stayed. I got home and couldn't sleep, I'm sure I wasn't the only one.

A day or two passed and I went back hoping for a happier situation. Everyone was out of the initial shock, but the mood wasn't much better. Casey had decided to finally go home. She was going to bring one person with her to be there to comfort her, to be there to listen to her, to be her shoulder to cry on. Out of everyone, I was picked. I was a little nervous not knowing what to expect, not knowing if I could be what she needed. Although, I agreed to do it hoping I had what it took to get her through the night.

We drove home with her dad who didn't live far from her house. The ride home was definitely nerve racking for everyone in the car. This was the first time Casey had left the hospital, so she was scared something might happen with Jeff and she wouldn't be there. We got home, and the house seemed empty. The dogs were excited to see her but sensed that something was wrong. We took her bags to her room, and she saw a glass jar labeled 365 things I love about you. She immediately burst into tears. I was bewildered on what was happening, I hadn't noticed that glimmer of the past, and I didn't realize how hard it would be for her to come home.

I just hugged her to let her know that I wasn't there to judge her, that I was there to support her. She put her things away and went into the closet and saw his clothes. I knew this would be hard. I just let her stare at them and I didn't rush her. After a couple minutes she went back to putting stuff away although, her mind wasn't thinking about putting stuff away but about him. She decided to take a shower. She was in the bathroom for around 30 minutes and I had no idea what to do. I played with the dogs, but I wasn't the one they wanted. I called my mom and told her that everything was ok, she told me to be strong for Casey. Those two small words came with lots of responsibility. Be strong.

I tried to be as much as possible, but the night was growing and as we became more and more tired, our bodies relaxed and we became sensitive. Every picture chipped a piece of our heart, every note, every little thing that had to do with Jeff hurt to look at. I know it was hard for me I can't imagine the pain Casey endured just being at the home they shared, with one part missing.

She walked out of the room into their office. I let her be in there alone for a few minutes then followed. She was crying reading the computer. I didn't realize what it was until I stepped closer to the screen. It was Caring Bridge, a website set up to update family and friends on the situation with Jeff, and people could leave comments. The things people were saying were breathtaking. She had no idea this many people cared about her and Jeff, she was getting love and hope and prayers from people she had only met once or twice and it was overwhelming for her, and hard to take in. We hugged once again and just held on.

It was time to go to bed and I knew it would take us both a while to fall asleep. She gave in to the dogs allowing them to sleep with us. I tried to lie down, though it was difficult with the dogs taking up most of the space on the bed. I would sleep on Jeff's side and her on her usual.

We laid there staring at the ceiling, gazing at something though not really looking at it. Too busy trying to comprehend the thoughts scrambling inside, I reached over and grabbed her hand. I wanted her to know that I was there to fill as much of the emptiness as possible, put some of the pieces of her heart back to where they belonged. But I knew I wasn't the one that could fill the hole she had. We both turned over and just eventually drifted off to sleep waking up every now and then, to grab the other's hand.

I hoped I had done the job I came to do, I knew I was there to help her, but in the end it helped me realize the love that we had, I knew from then on we could and would get through this.

Jessica, my cousin, was another person to spend the night with me. She is only two years younger than me, so we did a lot together growing up. She was working on her PhD at the time, and took a week off from school to comfort me. It meant a lot to me that she was there. This is how she recalled her sleepover.

During our childhood, Casey and I were much more than simply cousins, we were playmates, partners-in-crime, and, most of all, devoted pen pals. We would write about school, our friends, boys we liked, and our often annoying younger sibling. She was the keeper of all my most cherished secrets. However, as we got older, life seemed to get in the way. As schedules conflicted, our letters became less frequent. I cannot recall when we actually stopped writing each other, and it became only a memory we shared when reminiscing. While my love for Casey remained steadfast, I felt like the special bond that united us as young children had somehow faded. Things changed the day of Jeff's accident.

My mother called me the morning of June 25th and informed me that Jeff had been in an accident. She calmly tried to explain Jeff's condition with what little information she had at the time. Desperate for more details, I called several other family members. The general consensus was not good. Jeff had suffered a serious head injury and may not live. The only thing I could think of was Casey—my sweet cousin, my friend, my family, my pen pal. At that moment, nothing else mattered. I had to be with her.

The two and half hour drive to the hospital seemed to drag on for hours as thoughts, images, memories, and worries wrestled for my attention. As my younger sister and I walked into the hospital, I suddenly realized that I had not even called Casey to tell her that we were coming. In fact, I could not even remember the last time I had spoken to her; it had been several months for sure. What if she didn't want me there? What if it was awkward? What if I didn't know what to say? I wanted to tell her, "I am here. I love you. I don't care if you need to stay up crying all night long. I am here." But because I could not find the words, I vowed at that moment that I would let my actions speak for me.

In the days that followed, my role became quickly defined as the supportive gopher, Casey's personal assistant—always ready and waiting to fulfill any request. I would drive her to and from the hospital, direct traffic in the waiting room, supply the caffeine from the nearest Starbucks, run errands, wash clothes, etc. I was determined to alleviate at least some of Casey's pain and stress.

As I write this, my heart echoes the clouds of uncertainty and overwhelming feelings of pain and desperation, although moments later I am laughing out loud as I remember other times. Like when an indescribable stench woke me during my first sleepover night with Casey. I rolled over to face the other side of the bed desperate for clean air, but instead I found myself face-to-face with the culprit. The smell had come from Chicken, who was lying vertically on the bed next to me...upside down. Or, like when I had gone to the pet store for dog food early one morning to fuel Chicken's emissions. The bag was so large and heavy that I was forced to bend downward at the waist and shove the massive bag of food forward from the aisle to the checkout, a position that no self-respecting female should ever have to perform.

Amidst the tragedy, there came feelings of faith and hope. It is written that "all things work together for good to those who love God, to those who are called according to His purposes" (Romans 8:28). For my relationship with Casey, we were able to rekindle the special bond we shared so many years ago. For our family, and for Jeff, it was our refusal to ever let go of our love for one another that allowed healing and growth.

Unconscious Struggles

Journal update, Wednesday, June 29, 2011 (Written by Kristin, my cousin)

Last night, Jeff got a little restless and decided he didn't like the breathing tube, so he pulled it out. They got things back in order and had him resting well today. Because of the time that has lapsed, the doctors have decided it will be best to perform a couple of procedures that will be a bit more long term. 1. They are looking at inserting a Tracheotomy which will allow Jeff to breathe without the use of his nose or mouth. 2. They are looking at other options for feeding, one of which is a PEG tube, which is inserted into his stomach thru the abdominal wall. Both procedures are very common and should be completed with minimal complications. Casey went home last night for a nice home cooked meal from Tess and Brian, she visited with Buddie and Chicken then took some time for herself. She is coping with this in her own way. Casey knows that God is in control and although it is hard to understand it all, she has faith that God will take care of everything and it will work out the way he wants it to. We will keep you all updated as we have more information. Jeff's parents and all the family are grateful for everyone's support and prayers.

Although he was unconscious, Jeff moved around a lot. Pulling out his feeding and breathing tubes was a regular occurrence, so the option of having fewer tubes was a relief. He would get very agitated and would lift his upper body up off the bed. It was disturbing to watch him. He would lie there so still, his chest mechanically moving up and down with the rhythm of his breathing machine. Then, I would notice his fingers or toes start to twitch. That was my sign to get up because he was about to do something. Suddenly, with his eyes still closed, his head and chest would spring off the pillow, and his hand would rush to his face to pull on one of the many tubes protruding from it. The nurses had to restrain his arms, feet, and chest to keep Jeff from hurting himself.

Having Jeff restrained made him look even worse than he already did. Now added to the tubes and wires, his arms and legs were strapped to the bed. There was a mesh restraint around his chest, keeping him from rising up. Even with all the restraints, he would manage to get his hands to his face. Eventually, someone had to be stationed by his bedside twenty-four hours a day to prevent him from pulling his tubes out.

There were so many ups and downs throughout the process. It wasn't like Jeff had an accident, and then he gradually got better. One day, he would be a little better, and then the next he would take a step back. The day they did his tracheotomy was difficult because they had to completely sedate him to do it so that he couldn't move during the procedure. So that day, no progress was made. It felt like we put him a step back.

On top of that, I felt like I had given up hope that Jeff would wake up soon. I knew that the tracheotomy was easy to reverse, and they could simply pull the tube from his neck once he awoke. Somehow though, it still felt like I was giving in to the fact that he wouldn't wake up in the next few hours, or even days. I just had to trust that we were making the right decisions.

God gave me a lot of signs very early on to assure me that he was present and would not abandon me. The first couple of signs were comic relief for me that provided a little comfort. People can say they were just coincidences, but I trust that God's hand was in everything. On our anniversary, just a few weeks before Jeff's accident, I gave Jeff a jar with 365 love messages. Some of them were thoughtful and romantic, some were comical, and others were just famous phrases about love and marriage. I brought it to the hospital to read to him each day.

The very first one that I pulled out to read said, "Love is like a perpetual anesthesia." There was Jeff, lying unconscious in the bed in front of me. I thought, *He must love me a lot!*

The next day, the message said, "I hope you know CPR because you make my heart stop." All the messages were tightly folded up and packed into a small jar. There was no way to see the message before it was taken out and unfolded. Out of all the 365 messages in that jar that I could have pulled out, those were the two that were selected.

Before the accident, I had been reading a book that was all about prayer. I hadn't opened it in a few days before Jeff's accident. When I finally did attempt to read again, I opened this book, and the bookmark was sitting at the beginning of the next chapter that was titled, "Seek the God of the Impossible in Illness."[2] It discussed how to pray when you or a loved one was sick. I actually remember the last time I was reading the book; I got to this chapter and stopped. I thought, *Well, that's going to be a boring chapter. I don't know anyone who is sick.* I almost skipped over it, but instead, I placed the bookmark, put it down, and forgot all about it. God knew when I would open it again, and that it would apply exactly to my situation.

Later, I had been talking to a friend on the phone about the signs that were being presented to me. When I hung up, I went to the living room, and my cousin, Jessica, was staying with me that night. She had no idea what I'd been talking about, but she had a verse that she wanted to read me. It was, "Therefore, do not worry about tomorrow, for tomorrow will worry about itself. Each day has enough trouble of its own" (Matthew 6:34). It was like God was telling me he knows what I'm going through, and he will take care of me. I had no control over the situation, and I needed to give my worries to him. God was reminding me that he was big enough to take care of everything; I wasn't.

On the nights that I did go home in those first weeks after the accident, my mom was one of the people to stay with me. My parents divorced when I was very young, and growing up, I lived with my mom. We have gone through many trials together, and she knows how I react in difficult circumstances. We spent many late nights talking about life. We have passed the point now where she feels like she has to parent me and have crossed over into more of a friendship. I value her opinion much more now than when I was younger. She was one of the few I shared some of my deeper hurts and worries with during this journey. She shared her thoughts with me from that night.

> I'll never forget that first sleepover with Casey after the accident. Not only were we greeted by a very excited Buddie and a tail-wagging Chicken, but on every table in the house there were notes of encouragement and expressions of love from their neighbor Tess. On the kitchen table sat a warm home-cooked meal, and sitting squarely in the middle of their bed was a Teddy Bear the size of a ten year old child. It had a note pinned to its chest; I don't remember the exact words, but I'm sure Casey does, and I'm also sure that bear shared a spot with Buddie and Chicken on the bed next to Casey in the months that followed.
>
> We talked a little bit that night, but Casey was exhausted in every way possible, so we went to bed, or should I say, tried to find a comfortable spot next to the

> Great Dane without rolling over on Buddie. As I lay there, I was thankful for Tess's gesture. It had to be hard for Casey to walk into that house without Jeff. Love and laughter lived there, along with their hopes and dreams. There were no dreams that night, only the nightmare that Jeff might never come home to this house again, or for that matter, ever wake up again.
>
> The next morning, Casey thought she was ready to face the financial implications of the accident and see if she could get an extension on some of their bills. Moments later, after trying to explain her situation to several inconsiderate and incompetent customer service representatives…her dam of strength and courage finally gave way to waves of grief.
>
> As a mother, you say and do what you can to bring comfort, but it's just not enough. What I remember most throughout that day was how I longed for yesterday's troubles…the worries at work, bills to pay, silly disagreements, weight gain! It hit me like a ton of bricks that the troubles of yesterday were what the book "Don't Sweat the Small Stuff" was all about. When your loved ones are in pain, or may never recover, nothing else matters. *Nothing else matters.* I took so much for granted…the pure simple joy of getting up each morning, the ability to go to work, to pay bills, to love and be loved, and the importance of family. In one split second, tragedy slaps you in the face and teaches you one of life's most difficult lessons…Live each day to the fullest, love one another, and truly, don't sweat the small stuff.

The Friday after the accident (almost a week) was the first day that I was not at the hospital first thing in the morning. It was time to figure out how I was going to pay bills and see if I could get an extension on any of them. I didn't realize how hard that would be. It was just a few bills. The first call I made was to suspend Jeff's cell phone. The cheerful customer service representative answered after a few rings and asked how she could help me.

"I need to suspend my husband's line," I told her.

"How long would you like to suspend it for? We can do a temporary suspension, or we can terminate the line," she explained.

How long? I thought. I didn't know how long. *Terminate the line?* I didn't want to get rid of it completely; he was going to wake up! Suddenly, emotions flooded my mind. "He's been in an accident. He's unconscious right now, and I don't know when he's going to wake up," I blurted out, then started crying. Through sobs, I continued, "We lost his phone when he had his accident, and I just don't want someone else using it. I don't want to get rid of his line because I want him to wake up."

I can imagine the representative on the other end sitting there with her mouth open, not knowing what to say to my emotional outburst. I apologized as I took a few minutes to cry while she did her best to help me. I was overwhelmed with how difficult it was to make such a simple phone call. All I had to do was turn Jeff's phone off, but that simple task brought to reality many of the questions that I didn't want to ask. How long would he be unconscious? Would he ever wake up? Would he be able to even use a phone again if he did wake up?

I had to make several more phone calls that morning, and I cried through almost every one of them. It got easier toward the end, but each call brought up more questions, more emotions. Not to mention, I had no idea at that point when or if I was even going to be able to pay the bills in the future.

When I finally got to the hospital, it was around lunchtime. While I was on the way, his mom called me and said that he was making facial expressions for the first time! Of course, the one day that I'm not there, he starts doing exciting new things! When I got there, he had just thrown up, and the nurses were trying to clean him. Then they had to replace his feeding tube. It took almost two hours before they finally let me in to see him. I was going crazy in the waiting room. It was the longest amount of time I'd been away from him since his accident, and it hadn't exactly been an easy morning. It was torture! It was worth the wait though, when I was finally allowed back in the room to see him and his funny new expressions.

Another struggle the doctors had with Jeff was keeping him comfortable versus allowing him to wake up. Jeff would squirm and become very agitated; he was in visible pain. When this happened, it was usually when he tried to pull his tubes out. Because of that, the nurses often had to increase the dose of sedatives they were giving him to keep Jeff comfortable. However, by doing this, it made it harder for him to wake up on his own. They would often decrease the level of sedatives and keep a close eye on him to see if he would wake up. But then, he would become a danger to himself, and they would be forced to increase them again.

Watching Jeff agitated and fighting his restraints was really difficult. I could tell that he was in pain and uncomfortable, but there was nothing I could do about it. Either the doctors had to increase his medications to keep him comfortable, or allow him to suffer to offer him the chance to wake up. It was aggravating. I wanted him to be able to wake up, but I also didn't want him to have to suffer and be uncomfortable. The best thing I could do was to just trust the doctors.

I had some people tell me that I needed to do research, talk to other doctors, and make sure I knew exactly what the doctors were doing because they could make mistakes or have a different viewpoint than I had. I understood where those people were coming from, but I didn't know anything about brain injuries. I didn't know what was best. Jeff was at one of the best head injury facilities in the country, so I chose to trust the doctors.

I didn't just blindly let them do anything they wanted; I did ask a ton of questions. It helped to have a notepad that I carried with me. I would write down any questions that I thought of if a doctor wasn't there to ask. I could also write down the answers. There was so much information to remember that I found myself asking the same questions over and over again. I made sure that I understood, to the best of my ability, what the doctors were doing and why. If I disagreed with something, I would ask more questions and give my opinion. Other than that, I trusted their judgment.

While I did trust the doctors, I wanted to make sure their orders were being followed correctly. After shift changes, I always made sure that the new nurses understood how to take care of Jeff. I checked to make sure they were washing out his mouth so he didn't get an infection from the ventilator. I verified that they were turning him every two hours to prevent bedsores. I learned how to read all the monitors and checked that he was receiving the correct dose of medications. I learned what all the different beeps and alarms meant, so I knew when to be worried and when something just needed to be refilled. Looking back now, I'm sure those nurses loved having someone constantly peeking over their shoulders.

It was a running joke that by the time Jeff got out of there, I could be a doctor because I was keeping myself so informed. Jeff was at a teaching hospital. Therefore, many of his nurses were very new. There would be times when I was able to tell them what an alarm meant or what needed to be done before they were able to figure it out. There was one nurse that seemed particularly inexperienced. One of Jeff's feeding tube alarms started beeping to indicate it needed to be refilled. Her eyes got wide, and she started searching around for the source of the alarm. I told her what it was, and she immediately calmed down. She informed me that it was her first day, and she was nervous.

We found that it would help Jeff to have something in his hands to grab and play with. It kept him occupied and seemed to keep him from fidgeting with his tubes as much. So we would roll up washcloths and let him hold them in his hands. One time, we had only given him one, and he started to play with it. He would toss it almost like he was trying to get it to his other hand. However, his hands were tied down, so he couldn't throw it very far. It usually landed on his stomach, so I would pick it up and give it back to him. He did this several times before I stopped picking it up. Then he continued to toss it, but when I wouldn't get it for him, he started trying to get it himself. He would pull on his blanket until he got the cloth close enough to grab. Then he would do it again. It was wonderful to see that he was able to problem solve! This was the first sign of cognitive functioning.

I stayed at the hospital as much as our family would allow me to. We took turns staying overnight, sleeping in the waiting room. I went home every other night to get some rest in a real bed, but it was so hard to go. I was so afraid that he would wake up, and I wouldn't be there. However, we weren't allowed to stay in Jeff's room overnight; we had to stay in the waiting room. But at least in the waiting room, the nurse could come get me if something happened, or if he woke up.

After about a week, everyone was trying to get me to agree not to have anyone stay overnight. That was extremely difficult for me. I understood why everyone else thought it was all right. They all had spouses and/or children to go home to. They had a life outside of the hospital. I didn't.

Jeff is my life; we have no children. I went home to a house with my dogs but with no husband. It was lonely. I couldn't sleep well at home because I was so worried about what was going on at the hospital. It was easier for me to just sleep in the waiting room. I was afraid he would wake up, and not only would I not be there, but no one would. I didn't understand why they wouldn't just let me stay every night. It was frustrating and irritating. I felt like we were abandoning him. Jeff was all I had, and they wanted me to leave him!

No one seemed to understand the difference between being his wife and being someone else close to him. Everyone else left the hospital and had someone to go home to and find comfort. I had no one at home to console me. I had no one to take care of me. My companion was lying unconscious in a hospital bed. Yes, friends and family took turns coming home with me, but it wasn't the same. Everyone else would eventually be able to walk away. They would go back to their lives, go back to their families. No matter how bad it was for them now, they would eventually go home and resume life as normal. I would bear the everyday twenty-four-hour burden of taking care of my husband long after the physical wounds healed and after everyone else stopped noticing Jeff's deficits.

WAKING UP

> Journal update, Saturday, July 2, 2011
>
> He opened his eyes! It was for just a couple minutes, but he opened them. He looked around, he looked at me, he looked at the doctors in the room, then back at me, and he watched me for a minute. He closed them, and we asked him to open them again, and he did! He squeezed the nurse's hand on command. He wasn't able to give a thumbs up, but this is the biggest news for me so far! He is back to sleeping again now. So, we are making progress. Before I left for the evening, Jeff opened his eyes again. The nurse asked if he was in pain, and he shook his head no. He was able to lift two fingers when we asked him to. This is the best day we have had since the accident! I'm so excited! This is the first step of many down the long road we are about to take, but we have started moving.

I wrote that update on my cell phone, it was difficult to go into much detail then, so let me do it now. There were two nurses in the room with me. One was on either side of the bed. I was helping them turn Jeff over so he didn't develop bedsores. As they did, his eyes flashed open like they often did when he was in pain, but this time was different. He didn't have the empty look that he always had before. His eyes focused! He looked at me, then over to the nurse on his right side. He looked back at me and furrowed his brows as if to say, "Who is that?"

"His eyes are open!" I shouted. "Jeff, you have been in an accident. You are in the hospital." I told him as my eyes began misting. He closed his eyes again. About that time, the nurses remembered to start testing to see if he could follow commands.

They yelled at him, "Jeff! Open your eyes!" and he did again!

The nurse next to me put Jeff's fingers around her hand. "Squeeze my hand, Jeff!" He did it!

"Jeff! Make a 'thumbs-up' sign!" she said. He didn't do it, so I started asking him to do it, but he closed his eyes again. We asked him to open them, but he didn't this time. Then suddenly, his left arm shot straight out to his side; he put his thumb in the air, then retracted it as quickly as he put it out there. It was like he was saying, "There, are you happy?"

He went back to sleep for a few more hours. My sister Kelby was in the room with me, and we were going to leave soon. The nurses were performing one of their hourly neurological exams.

"Jeff! Jeff, can you hear me? Open your eyes if you can hear me!" one of the nurses shouted. He was able to open them again. This time they were ready to test his neurological functioning.

"Are you in pain?" she asked. At first, he didn't respond; then, he shook his head no. They asked him to do a few commands that he was unable to perform. He was able to lift two fingers before he fell back to sleep.

After eight days of being unconscious, Jeff finally opened his eyes! And it wasn't just because he was in pain. He opened them on his own and looked around. He was aware. This was a miracle. This was the first real sign of hope for me. I knew that God was with me the whole time; I knew that he would take care of us, but this was the first time that I was excited and hopeful about the future. Jeff wasn't going to live the rest of his life in a coma; he was going to wake up.

I need to explain what it means to "wake up" from a coma. It's not like in the movies where the person opens their eyes, and they are instantly better. It is a very slow process. It can look different for everyone. Sometimes the person can begin therapy and respond to commands before the eyes open. With Jeff, the first sign was him opening his eyes. Like the journal entry said, it was just for a few seconds. Then, he went back to sleep for several hours and opened his eyes again for a few seconds.

Over the next few days, he would open his eyes for longer, and it would happen more frequently. Even when Jeff had his eyes open, he was still not fully awake. Doctors have different opinions on when the person is actually awake, but just because a person's eyes are open does not mean they have woken up. Because of the differing opinions, I am not exactly sure when Jeff woke up in the medical sense. I just know that opening his eyes was the first sign for us that he was beginning that process.

Kelby, my sister, and I were standing by Jeff's bed after he closed his eyes when all of a sudden, she looked down and saw water pooling at our feet. At first, we thought it was coming from one of his IV bags. Then we realized that it was coming from the toilet in the room! It had overflowed and was beginning to flood the entire room. That was our cue to leave for the evening because they had to switch Jeff to a different room!

Kelby stayed with me that night. She drove me home, and the whole way I was on the phone, calling people to tell them the good news about Jeff opening his eyes. This was the most excited I had been in a long time. I remember when I finally got off the phone I just sat there, soaking it in. I just couldn't believe that he was finally coming around. After eight days of waiting, eight days of wondering if he would wake up, eight days of agony, torture, and uncertainty, I can't convey the amount of excitement, joy, and peace I had at that moment. I also realized that I must have been yelling with excitement when I was on the phone because it was suddenly very quiet in the car. I looked over at Kelby, and she had a grin on her face.

That was the first night at home when I didn't cry myself to sleep. Instead of sulking into the house and falling into bed, there was excitement and laughter. That year, I was doing what I called the 365-Day Project. I took a picture every day for a year and posted it online. So that night, Kelby took a picture of my eye to post, representing Jeff opening his eyes.

I knew that Jeff's recovery was going to be a long process, but at this point, I still had not grasped what that all meant. He had just opened his eyes, so in my mind, everything was going to be just fine. Different social workers kept talking to me about therapy. I was in denial about Jeff needing therapy early on. In my head, I still pictured him waking up and coming home. I thought that the long recovery process would happen at home. I never imagined that he would spend months in different rehabilitation hospitals.

I was told again and again that he would need therapy, but it just wasn't sinking in. I pictured his recovery would involve learning who people were again and other memory problems. It never occurred to me that he would have to relearn the most basic functions that we so easily take for granted in our day-to-day living, such as eating or dressing.

Once Jeff started to awaken, I had so many more questions for the doctors. They said they would know more once he woke up. So I wanted those answers immediately. Yet, they still weren't able to give them. Once he began to awaken, they just told me that only time would tell how well he would get, and it would be around two years before he stopped making recovery.

However, they didn't know what that meant. Would he be close to how he was before, or would he never be able to be unsupervised? It was so maddening having so many worries and questions but not having any answers. I'm a planner; I wanted to know what Jeff's recovery would look like so I could plan out our lives accordingly. I didn't have a choice. Of course, much of the information they were giving me, I wasn't able to process. I was hearing what I wanted to hear much of the time. Only time would tell what the future would hold.

By Day 10, which was also the 4th of July, Jeff seemed to be making miraculous progress. Any time I tried to sit down to get something done, he would wake up. He began responding to yes and no questions and was following commands more consistently.

That morning, the nurse was trying to clean his mouth, and he wouldn't let her. He would purse his lips together and toss his head from side to side, like a toddler refusing medicine.

"Jeff, she is just trying to brush your teeth, she doesn't want to hurt you," I explained to him. "If you will let her clean your teeth, then I will give you a kiss."

He glared at me, but he did allow the nurse to clean his mouth. When she finished, he turned to me and puckered his lips!

I had to learn how to have patience with Jeff during his recovery process. Because many of the connections in his brain were severed, the messages his brain wanted to send had to find new routes. This took much longer than it used to. I would ask Jeff a question, and he would just stare back at me. So I would ask again or ask the question in another way. After about thirty to forty-five seconds, he would finally respond. It was taking that long for his brain to send messages. The responses were usually just yes or no since he wasn't able to talk at this point. It amazed me that something as simple as shaking his head could take so much time and effort.

When Jeff had his tracheotomy, they basically cut a hole in his throat and attached a breathing machine to it. However, there was a hole in the tube right in front of his neck that allowed room air to pass through. I'm not exactly sure what the hole was for, but it provided for some entertainment.

Jeff had pneumonia, so he was constantly coughing up mucus from his lungs. This little hole allowed that mucus to fly across the room. I learned this the hard way when I was standing in front of him and got a nice wad of it in my hair. I quickly learned that it was best to stand beside him, not in front of him, and to move quickly when I heard him start to cough.

My brother, Nick, and I have always had a very love-hate relationship. So, being the nice, considerate sister that I am, I told him that Jeff liked it when you stood at his feet. Fortunately for him, one of the nurses warned him what would happen. Luckily for me though, Jeff managed to cough right as Nick was walking in front of him! Nick did dodge out of the way, but it provided me with some comic relief. Another time, he managed to cough so hard that it went all the way across the room and landed on the nurse's keyboard!

Jeff was becoming much more animated. Any time I went home to sleep, I always returned to the hospital early enough to be there for the doctor's rounds. This is where I received the most information about Jeff's progress and what to expect that day. Most of the time, the mood was very somber. This morning, however, there were smiles and laughter.

I was standing just outside Jeff's room with the doctors while they discussed what the day would hold for Jeff. One of Jeff's sisters was in the room with him while I talked to the doctors. Jeff had to have these booties on his feet to help the circulation in his legs and feet since they had been non-ambulatory for so long. Every couple minutes, they would fill with air to compress, then release. Jeff hated them and was confused by them. Every time they would fill with air, he looked at his feet in confusion. He wasn't able to talk, but he conveyed this message with his many facial expressions.

The bed had been positioned so that Jeff was sitting up. His sister was stationed at his feet, and I could hear her laughing and telling Jeff no.

"Well, this is a nice change. I see smiles and hear laughter. What is going on in there?" one of the doctors commented as he peered over my shoulder into the room.

I turned around to see what the commotion was. Jeff was using his feet to kick off his booties. His sister was futilely trying to stop Jeff. Every time she would put them back on, Jeff would kick them off. His lips would curl into a grin of satisfaction every time he got them off; then, he would look at his sister as if to dare her to put them back on again. The doctors were very encouraged by the change in Jeff, as well as the mood in the room.

Beyond Words

On Day 11, Jeff was awake most of the day. At one point, we were alone together in the room, and I was standing next to his bed. Jeff brought my hand to his lips and kissed it. Later that day, I was leaving the room, and Jeff puckered his lips for a kiss. I reached down to kiss him and told him I love him. Then he mouthed back that he loves me too. They were such small acts, but it reminded me that my husband was in there somewhere. Beneath the crazy hair, dazed eyes, restraints, and tubes, my husband was there. The only way he knew how, Jeff was trying to show me that he hadn't left me.

I cannot express how relieved I was when Jeff did those things. All my fears about him not liking me anymore melted away. He recognized me; he knew who I was, and he loved me! I didn't have to worry about whether he would want me anymore. Of all the people that were in and out of his room, he chose to act that way around me.

In addition, he seemed to remember that we were married. I was wearing his wedding ring on a chain around my neck. I remember that he looked at his ring finger where his ring should have been, then looked at me with concern. I showed him the ring around my neck, and he seemed satisfied with that. My husband remembered me, remembered that we were married, and still loved me! I could now start to worry about all the other things the doctors had warned me about.

Things were really starting to look up at this point. It was easier to have hope since Jeff was doing better. This was a time full of excitement and celebrating small accomplishments. We were excited about everything that he was doing because it meant he was making progress. I was so encouraged because it seemed like God was answering each and every prayer that I asked people to pray for.

By this time, I was starting to be able to pray again. It was much easier to tell other people specifically what to pray for, but I was still having a difficult time doing it myself. I was able to utter short prayers. I continued to struggle with it nonetheless, not knowing how to pray in such a situation.

Jeff still had to be restrained during this time. Even though he was more awake, he was not conscious enough to understand what was going on. I would tell him that he had a tube in his nose and not to bother it, and he would nod as if he understood. Then a few seconds later, he would try to pull it out. If he did understand what I expressed, he was incapable of remembering that I had informed him of it.

One thing that helped me get through all this was laughing about it. In addition to having his hands tied down, Jeff also required mittens on his hands. He was determined to get his hand to his face to pull the tubes out. No matter how tight his restraints were, Jeff weaseled his hand close enough to his face to get the tubes, so the mitts made it a little more difficult once his hand got there. He hated the mitts. He would bring his hand up and hit them on his face, then give me this confused and irritated look as if to say, "Take these off!"

When one of us was in the room and could hold his hand, we could take the mitts off. There was one time when my dad and I were standing on his left side, and one of his sisters was standing on his right. We were both holding his hands. He kept acting like he wanted to scratch his nose, so she cautiously let him bring his hand to his face, making sure he wouldn't go for the tubes. He scratched his nose, then put his hand back down. Then he did it again, but while he was scratching, he felt the tube and yanked it out before we could do anything to stop him!

His sister jumped about a foot in the air, screamed bloody murder, and turned around. My dad and I rushed to stop him. The nurses dashed into the room to see what the commotion was all about. Once we had his hands again, we all started laughing. Jeff was satisfied to have gotten it so far out. Unfortunately though, the nurse had to shove it back in. He was not happy about that. I thought he would learn his lesson, but he proceeded to jerk it out several more times before we were finally able to leave it out.

Later that same day, the doctor came in and removed Jeff's tracheotomy. Just like that…he came in the room, said it was time for it to come out, and pulled it right out of his neck! It took Jeff a while to figure out how to move air around the gaping hole in his neck, but he began trying to talk to us. The first intelligible words that he said were directed at me: "I love you."

Otherwise, he kept trying to communicate, but we weren't able to understand most of what he said. He would make these funny facial expressions when we didn't get it. I thought he was frustrated because we couldn't understand what he was saying. However, as he learned to push the air around the hole, I learned that the words that he was saying were gibberish. When he couldn't find the words he wanted to say, he just made them up.

Around the same time, the doctors wanted Jeff to start sitting up. Because he had been lying down for so long, Jeff was not able to sit up on his own. The nurses would adjust his bed so it allowed him to sit up with his feet hanging down, almost like he was in a chair. They wanted him to get used to being in that position before they moved forward to helping him stand. I recall being so happy that he was sitting up, but at the same time, I felt bewildered and confused.

There was Jeff, sitting up in his bed, with his glasses on. He was slouched over and leaning on his left side. He could barely hold his head up. When he looked around the room, he was very sluggish. He reminded me of someone that was inebriated and had a "deer in the headlights" look. He didn't seem to have a sense of where he was but also seemed blissfully content and irritated at the same time. He had no clue what we had all been through or that there was really anything wrong with him. I was so happy that he was making progress but confused about being happy that my husband looked and acted that way.

The next day was a big one for Jeff. He was finally cleared to move out of the ICU and into the general ward. While it was exciting that he was well enough for this move, the new level of care was not what I had hoped.

This night was a nightmare. By this time, I had been talked into not having anyone stay overnight with Jeff since they weren't letting us stay in the room with him anyway. When Jeff was moved from the ICU to the general ward, the doctors and nurses did not communicate with one another. They wouldn't let him have anything to eat or drink, and they did not understand that someone needed to be by his bedside at all times to keep him from pulling his tubes out.

When they finally did get someone in there, it was a kid who had no idea what was going on and had to keep leaving to ask questions or get someone to help him. Jeff was incredibly uncomfortable because they did not communicate the pain medications that he was on. He was usually agitated, but I had never seen him this bad. I ended up staying awake with him all night.

I was there with Jeff all alone; everyone else had gone home for the night. I was so afraid that he was not being treated properly. No one was communicating with one another, and I needed to speak with a doctor, but the nurses wouldn't get one for me. They kept telling me that a doctor had been paged, but no one would come. Around 1:00 or 2:00 a.m., I finally broke down and called my Aunt Sheila. I felt bad calling so late, but I didn't know what else to do. Her husband, who was a neurologist, was a huge help through this entire process, and I hoped they would know what to do.

I cried into the phone and explained what was going on. She had me go to the nurse's station and get a phone number for her. I don't remember now what it was for, and I don't know what she said when she called it, but a doctor finally came to see me shortly after. I explained what had transpired through the night and that Jeff was much more agitated than normal. It turned out that Jeff was unable to figure out how to urinate on his own, and his catheter had been removed. Minutes after it was reinserted, he calmed down significantly.

After that night, I knew that I had to get him out of the general ward and into a rehab hospital. So, I arranged for him to be moved that morning. However, I had to be gone most of the day to fill out paperwork for Jeff's disability income. I wanted to be at the hospital to make sure everything went smoothly with the transition to the new hospital.

I managed to get there just as the ambulance was taking him. I got to ride with him to the new hospital. He had to be sedated to keep him from moving around too much in the ambulance. I remember walking down the hall with the EMS team pushing him on the stretcher. He was awake and had this dazed look on his face. He seemed really astonished but was excited at the new scenery. He hadn't been outside of a hospital in two weeks. I can't imagine what he must have been thinking when that sun hit his face.

Beginning Rehabilitation

Journal update, Thursday, July 7, 2011

Sorry this update is so late; it was a very long day today. We had a lot of trouble getting Jeff discharged from the hospital. However, now he is at the rehab hospital and is loving it! They took all of his tubes and IVs out and put him in what looks like an adult playpen (called a Posey). We gave him some toys, and he sat up in bed and was having a great time. The facility has been generous enough to give us a private suite with an extra bed so I or another family member can be with him at all times. He is much happier here so far. PT did come see Jeff at the hospital this morning and had him stand and sit in a chair for about forty minutes. He wasn't able to hold himself up standing and wasn't able to walk, but he was able to sit up on his own!

So glad the move went well and a new chapter has begun! May God be with you both in the days ahead as Jeff regains his strength! So anxious to see him up and about…God is good! All the time!

Lynda Dinsdale

Recovery in the ICU, or in the hospital, was very unlike recovery in a rehabilitation hospital. The goals were different; therefore, everything was different. We were no longer worried about whether Jeff would live; the concern became recovery and relearning tasks that before had been second nature. There were still ups and downs, but they were different. Now I was more worried about long-term issues and whether I would be able to adjust to my new husband.

Contentment shined from Jeff's face. It was the first time that he seemed like he was comfortable. The tubes and machines were gone, and he was able to move freely. Sitting "Indian Style" in his bed, Jeff showed us that he had learned to sit up on his own. Jeff seemed happier, and I felt more comfortable once he was at the rehab hospital. The ICU did a great job while he was unconscious, but now that he was more alert, he needed a different type of care.

The staff at this hospital really seemed to understand that. They also let a family member stay in the room with him twenty-four hours a day. It made me feel so much better to know that someone could be with him anytime he needed something. I didn't have to worry that he was going to wake up in the middle of the night, wondering why he was alone.

Jeff was making progress in just the first day of being in rehab. His therapists allowed him to put his own shirt on with minimal help. He was able to get out of bed, stand up almost completely on his own, and even take a couple wobbly steps. Other than his balance being off a little, he did great. He was even able to put his arms around me and give me a hug! This was the first hug I had received from him since his accident! I was standing in front of Jeff, ready to catch him if he fell. He looked at me for a second, then reached his arms out, wrapped them around me, and pulled me in close. Tears welled in my eyes as I realized Jeff was communicating with me the only way he could.

One of the objectives of that first day was to have a formal swallow test done to see if Jeff could eat whole foods instead of the shakes they had been feeding him. Jeff's first experience with a formal swallow test was both frustrating and entertaining. What should have taken about twenty minutes, took about two hours, and we weren't even able to complete it!

In order to eat solid foods, Jeff had to chew and swallow different textured foods while undergoing an X-ray of his throat to make sure it was going down properly. The first obstacle was getting Jeff into a wheelchair to roll him downstairs. Jeff's room was on the second floor of the hospital, while the X ray machine was on the first. At first, Jeff didn't even want to get out of the bed. When he did, he was so excited about standing that he didn't want to sit down. He didn't like the wheelchair at all and refused to sit in it. There was a large reclining chair next to his bed for his visitors to sit in, and he thought it looked more comfortable, so that's where he sat. Fortunately, the chair had wheels on it. So, we decided we would just roll him around in that instead of the wheelchair.

We began the journey to the elevator, and every few feet, Jeff would put his feet down and try to stand up. I had to walk in front of the chair, holding Jeff's feet up to keep him from getting out. If we tried to bring up the footrest, he just kicked it back down, thinking it was a game. He was captivated by his changing surroundings. He kept looking around and grinning. Despite everything that was happening, he seemed very happy.

Once we finally maneuvered him downstairs and into the X-ray room, we had to try to get him to sit in another chair because his big recliner didn't fit in the X-ray machine. It was an impossible task, and Jeff refused to get out of his chair. The therapists decided to attempt to get his chair to fit in the machine. It did, but just barely. Jeff had to sit in the perfect position for the X-ray to take pictures of his throat. Again, Jeff did not want to cooperate with us. He wanted to sit forward.

After about an hour of trying, Jeff was getting irritated, and so were we. We finally decided that this was not going to happen, and we would try again on Monday. We began the long journey back through the hallways and up the elevator, with me carrying Jeff's legs in front of him the whole way. He was pleased to be back in his room and crawled right back into bed. We zipped him up in the Posey, and all breathed a sigh of relief.

There were many moments at this facility when I was completely overwhelmed. There was my husband, lying in his Posey, which was basically a playpen. He wore a diaper because he was unable to control his bodily functions. This was one of the hardest adjustments to make.

Because Jeff was in a Posey, the nurses didn't want him to have any tubes that he could pull out of himself, but he was still unable to use the restroom. His problem wasn't that he was unable to hold it, but that his brain didn't send the signals that he needed to go. Therefore, every few hours, I had to help the nurses hold him down while they inserted a catheter to relieve his bladder and then remove it again. It was extremely painful for Jeff, and it took at least four people to hold him down.

He would squirm, try to hit or bite us, and yell obscenities at us, anything to make us stop. The alternative was having him remove a more permanent type of catheter himself and cause damage. Normally, this would be done by nurses, without my help. However, my voice seemed to be the only thing that kept him even remotely calm. It killed me to see the look of hurt and betrayal in his eyes. I was supposed to be the one protecting and helping him. Instead, I was holding him down while the nurses hurt him. Thankfully, now he has no memory of those torturous moments.

He was unable to bathe himself, so I helped the nurses change him and give him sponge baths. He was incapable of walking, talking coherently, or feeding himself. He was, in all practical senses, a baby. My thirty-one-year-old husband, the man who I was supposed to spend the rest of my life with, who I was supposed to have babies with, was a baby himself. It was a running joke in our family before the accident, that when people asked why we didn't have children, I would say, "I already have one," and point to Jeff. But this wasn't a joke. This wasn't Jeff just acting immature; this was reality.

Mothers are wired to care for their children. Mothers are designed to care for their children. Wives are not wired or designed to care for their husbands as though they are children. Husbands and wives were designed to help each other, to share in the burdens, to be partners. The Lord God said, "It is not good for the man to be alone. I will make a helper suitable for him" (Genesis 2:18). God didn't say he would make a caregiver for him. That didn't seem to matter anymore though. I was going to be a mother to my husband, at least for now, and although I wanted to have children someday, this was not what I pictured.

During this stage of Jeff's recovery, he had a lot of hallucinations. We had to let him rest a lot, not just because he was tired, but because his brain was on overload. He would be talking to us and then start talking to someone that wasn't in the room. So when he had a lot of visitors, it was extra distracting to him. For him, there weren't just two visitors in the room, there might be several. We let him have a lot of time by himself, and he would seem very content talking to himself. Using the toys he had in the bed as a phone was also a fun pastime for him, bringing the toys to his face and having a conversation with someone he believed to be on the other end.

It was oddly relaxing to watch him do this. I knew it wasn't normal, but he seemed so happy talking to these people that weren't there. I was relieved to know that he wasn't in pain, and he was enjoying himself. Even though he was zipped up into his Posey, in a hospital, unable to do anything for himself, he was content. He was blissfully unaware of the stresses of life, and the torture that I was being dragged through. It calmed me to see him so stress-free.

Laughter and Hope

> The last time I saw you and Jeff at James and your Mom's house he was sneaking the candy from the piñata to you, I was thinking about how sweet and funny he was. Asking you what you wanted him to get next and telling you not to trade his favorite candy with the other kids while he was gone. You are a perfect couple and I know he feels blessed to have you there for him through all of this. May God continue to heal Jeff fully and also continue to be a strength for you as Jeff's support line. Love to you both!
>
> —Bill and Pat Hermes

Throughout our journey, we searched for ways to laugh. Laughter provided a break from the constant stresses. It brought hope that more joys would come in the future. Obviously, there was a lot to cry about, but we were able to make light of our impossible situation. Jeff was such a light-hearted guy that sometimes he made it impossible not to laugh at him. It also reminded me of who he was before.

Another stage that Jeff was going through, which no one prepared me for, was his fascination with being naked. For whatever reason, Jeff went through a few days where he didn't want to wear clothes! I would work so hard with the therapists to get him dressed; then, he would take everything back off again. While we were happy to see that he was able to do this on his own, it was disheartening to see that he preferred his birthday suit. There were several therapy sessions that Jeff did without pants on. I was so embarrassed for him, but all the therapists were great about it and said it was a common occurrence. We just had to teach him that he has to wear clothes when other people are around.

Unfortunately, this wasn't just with his therapists, it was with everyone. One day, my mom was coming for a visit, and I couldn't get Jeff to put his clothes on! She arrived, and I had just gotten him dressed, so I went to the door to let my mom in. When I turned back around, he had already undressed himself again! I tried a couple of times until we just decided that we would pull the curtain, and I would visit with my mom on the other side of the room. Thankfully, this stage only lasted a couple of days.

By day 15, Jeff was already standing and walking some on his own. He was still pretty uncoordinated, but he was getting the concept. He was even able to play catch with his therapist. It was like teaching a child to catch a ball. His reaction was very slow, so by the time he realized the ball was coming to him and closed his hands, it had already fallen to the ground.

Conversation was beginning to make more sense, but Jeff had a lot of difficulty finding the right words. Wanting to say one thing, something completely different would come out. Some crazy things came out too. One time, he just randomly told me that he put grandma in the fire, and she got hot. He was able to say phrases that were familiar to him a lot easier than he was able to string a sentence together. His humor seemed to be returning.

Once he was able to get out of the bed to shower, he needed help with balance and remembering what to do. So every day an occupational therapist would come in and help him with his shower. One morning, his therapist, a very large, muscular guy, was helping Jeff get dressed. He handed Jeff his deodorant and asked if he knew where it went. Jeff looked at him and said, "Bend over. I'll show you." I was waiting for the therapist to smack him, or something, but he remained very calm and just played along.

Journal update, Sunday, July 10, 2011

> During therapy this morning, Jeff put his shirt on all by himself. It's inside out, but he did it on his own. We were going to try to get him to stand to look at some pictures, but he decided he wanted to go exploring instead. He saw that the bathroom door was open, so he went in, got in the shower, and started pulling on things. We had to call for help to get him back to the bed because he didn't give us time to get his safety belt on and wouldn't let us hold him. He was very wobbly and would lose his balance, so we had to keep our arms around him whether he wanted us to or not. Other than that, he was walking well. He very much has a mind of his own. Then, when we got him back to the bed, we were trying to get him to sit down, and he said he was going to sing for us. He started bobbing his head and bending his knees like he was dancing, but he made no music. It was pretty funny.
>
> Later in the day he was able to leave his room and walk around the hallway and down to the gym! He did a couple leg exercises in the gym. When we were walking, he would stop every couple of feet to give me a hug and kiss. It was really sweet. He is continuing to make more sense when he talks and is following commands better. The nurse came in a few minutes ago and asked Jeff his name, and he was able to tell her!

As I have said earlier, I had pictured a very different recovery process in my head. It didn't matter how much the doctors tried to prepare me, I was not able to grasp the depth of the recovery Jeff would experience. Jeff's entire brain was affected. Therefore, he needed to relearn everything. And I mean everything. I was there as he learned how to sit in a chair, figure out how to make his legs support him as he tried to stand up, walk, talk, chew, swallow, and bring food to his mouth to feed himself. He even had to relearn how to use the restroom. This wasn't just potty training like you would teach a toddler. Jeff's brain wasn't even getting the signals that his bladder was full. He had to relearn the signals that told him that his bladder was full.

This was going to take much longer than I ever expected it to. I was going to watch my husband grow up. I was going to see him go through the stages of infancy, toddlerhood, childhood, adolescence, and hopefully adulthood once again. I had to be patient because there was no way to rush him. I had been told many times, this is a marathon, not a sprint. There was no magic pill to give him (although later, Jeff would ask for one many times). There was no fast track to recovery, no easy way through. I would endure, with Jeff, the meticulously slow process of recovery.

Jeff celebrated his 32nd birthday on day 17 after his accident. It was another exciting day because he was approved to eat whole foods. So he was able to celebrate with a brownie. We were able to have a few family members over to have a small party in Jeff's room at the rehab hospital.

As I said before, it was easier for Jeff to say phrases that he knew than it was to string a sentence together. At his party, he was fiddling with the sheets in his bed, and my Aunt Sheila and cousins were getting ready to leave and asked him to give them a hug. He looked at them and said, "Uno momento, por favor." We all looked at each other, checking to see if we all heard the same thing, and then burst into laughter. Jeff couldn't string a sentence together in English, but apparently, he could speak Spanish!

I did have mixed emotions about his party. Jeff was at a stage where he was playing with infant toys. It provided the stimulation that he needed at that time. Still, it was very difficult to go shopping for infant toys to give to my thirty-two-year-old husband for his birthday. I walked into a store by our house to find a gift for my husband, then strolled to the baby/infant section of the store. I didn't expect to find myself there for a few more years, especially not to buy something for my husband. I browsed the toys and finally selected a few that would be useful for him in the recovery process.

The Power of Prayer

> Journal update, Tuesday, July 12, 2011
>
> This morning, I was reading Jeff some of the comments that people have left for us online, and he said, "That's a lot of prayers." He's right; we have so many people praying, and we are very thankful for it. I've been reading this book about prayer, and one of the chapters was about praying for the impossible. God answers prayers, as we have already seen. Jesus tells us to ask and we will receive and that we don't receive because we don't ask. I don't want to miss out on a miracle because I didn't ask. God can work miracles, and he can do things that are impossible for us. So, I'm not just praying for a speedy recovery, I'm praying for a miraculous recovery, a recovery that can only be explained by a miracle from God and not from anything we could have done. I'm praying that Jeff is just going to recover 100 percent overnight. I know this is impossible by our standards, but not by God's. I don't know if that is part of his plan or if he wants us to go down this long road. But I'm not going to miss a miracle like that because I didn't ask. I know he can say no; I know it may not be his plan, but please join with me in this prayer. Our God is the God of the impossible, nothing is too difficult for him.

By this time, I was starting to work through my struggles with praying. I knew that I wanted God's will for our lives, but I also wanted Jeff to get better. So I began praying for an impossible miracle. I began praying that Jeff was going to miraculously wake up and be better, no more therapy needed. I was alone in the room with him, so I sat down on his bed and placed my hands on his back. He was sitting up, playing with a toy.

I prayed out loud, "Lord, I have already seen you work miracles for Jeff. I know that you are the God of the impossible. I know that you can work impossible miracles so big that I can't even imagine them. I have been unsure how to pray, but I don't want to miss out on a miracle from you just because I didn't ask. So, Lord, I'm asking. I'm asking that you completely restore Jeff to the husband and man that he was before this accident. Not only do I ask for him to be one hundred percent restored, I ask that it be done overnight. I pray that Jeff will wake up and be healed. I pray that he will no longer need therapy. I pray that he will go back to work at his previous job and be able to perform his duties without any lasting effects from his brain injury. I realize this is impossible. I realize that in human standards, this could never happen. But you are above our human standards, Lord. You can do what we deem impossible. So I pray that you do this. If that is not your will though, Lord, I pray that you give me the strength and wisdom that I need to get through this. In Jesus's name, I pray. Amen."

People say they want to see a miracle, but no one ever wants to go through a circumstance where they need one. "Miracles never happen outside the context of mystery and mess."[3] We were in both mystery and mess, so I was going to embrace the miracle I knew God was capable of performing.

I finally came to the realization that if I didn't ask, God wouldn't be able to answer that prayer. God can always say no to a request. So I began praying for God to perform miracle after miracle. I had already seen him perform tons of them, but I wanted him to keep working. I didn't care what the books, statistics, and doctors said; I wanted God to completely restore my husband to the man he was before the accident. Once I had prayed for all the miracles I wanted to see; then, I would pray that God's will be done.

I had to have the faith of Shadrach, Meshack, and Abednego. When faced with bowing down to an idol or being thrown in a fiery furnace of death, they trusted God. They said, "If we are thrown into the blazing furnace, the God we serve is able to deliver us from it, and he will deliver us from Your Majesty's hand. But even if he does not, we want you to know, Your Majesty, that we will not serve your gods or worship the image of gold you have set up" (Daniel 3:17).

I just love that story. They were three ordinary guys, doing what God wanted them to do. They knew it was against what the king had ordered, but they were not going to disobey God just to conform to what everyone else was doing. They stood up for what they believed in. They had faith that God would save them, *but even if he didn't*, they were going to stand firm in their beliefs. I had to pray to God and ask him for a miracle. I had to trust and believe that God would heal my husband. *But even if he didn't*, I had to trust that it was part of God's bigger plan, and he would give me the strength to endure it.

When I was praying, Jeff turned around and said, "What are you doing?" It was clear and not gibberish. My heart leapt. Did God just answer my prayer? Then, he was back to how he had been a few seconds ago. I took that as a sign. I knew God was listening. Even if he never performed my impossible miracle, he performed so many others.

Looking back, I believe he did perform that impossible miracle; it just took time. God answered every prayer that I have prayed for Jeff and his recovery down to very specific details that I requested. He may not have worked in my timing, but he worked in his timing. I prayed that specific problems we had dealt with before the accident would no longer be an issue, and he granted even those prayers. He answered very specific prayers that I prayed so that I could have no excuse to say that it was anything except for God's hand. There was no way it could be a coincidence or modern medicine or even great doctors. It could only be God.

I finally started praying regularly again. Though I still struggled with exactly how to pray, I found some great examples in the Bible of how people prayed during difficult times in their lives. When Mary, the mother of Jesus, got the news from the angel that she would give birth to the Messiah, she had to have been terrified. But despite her fear, she told the angel, "Behold, I am the servant of the Lord; let it be to me according to your word" (Luke 1:38, ESV). She knew that getting pregnant before marriage was going to cause her a lot of hardships even though she had done nothing wrong. Yet, she prayed for God's will.

Before Jesus was handed over to be crucified, he went before God and prayed, "My Father, if it is possible, may this cup be taken from me, yet not as I will but as you will" (Matthew 26:39). Jesus knew he was about to endure a lot of physical and emotional pain, and he didn't want to go through it. Even Jesus asked that he not have to endure the pain, but then asked that God's will be done.

"God will put us in circumstances and situations in order to teach us how to talk with him."[4] It seemed that was what he was doing here. I had no idea how to pray in a situation like this, and then God revealed the way. It took me awhile, but this is how I tried to pray: I prayed for my impossible miracle, but I also prayed that if it wasn't God's will, then he would give me the strength I required to get through whatever was ahead of me.

In her Bible study book, Anne Graham Lotz wrote this:

> I heard that a turkey and an eagle react differently to the threat of a storm. A turkey runs under the barn, hoping the storm won't come near. An eagle leaves the security of its nest, spreads it wings, and rides the air currents of the storm, knowing its wings and the air currents will carry it higher in the sky than it could soar on its own.[5]

In my situation, I could either curl up in a ball, cry, and wait for the worst to be over, or I could trust in God and let him take me places that I would never be able to go on my own. Life was scary and uncertain; I had no idea where God was going to take me. I had no idea what it was going to mean to follow him through this. I could either hide in the barn and hope everything would just pass me by, or I could ride the currents of the storm. I knew that if I hid, I was going to be a lot worse off than if I soared with God. He could take me farther than I could ever dream to go on my own. He could help me see what I was incapable of seeing on my own.

During this journey, my dad was one of my biggest supporters. He had a flexible work schedule so he was able to be at the hospital more than most. I called him many times to get a break from being at the hospital or to get out of the house once Jeff was home. Sometimes, he would just come to sit with me and let me complain.

Growing up, he was a huge spiritual influence in my life, even if I didn't realize it at the time. His habits made a huge impact on my spiritual life. For as long as I can remember, when I got up to get ready, he was always sitting in the living room on the couch or out on the back porch, reading the Bible and having his daily quiet time with God. It was part of his morning ritual. He probably doesn't realize it, but it made an impression on me.

It's one thing to make kids go to church every Sunday (which my parents made sure that I did), but it's another to be devoted to God in everyday life. His dedication to a quiet time with the Lord every single day prompted me to do the same. I may not be quite as dedicated, as I am not a morning person like my dad, but over the years, I have tried to take time out of each day to spend with God. Sometime after the accident, he shared his thoughts with me.

> The basic instinct of a parent is to protect your children. It doesn't matter if they are 6 months old or 26 years old, I don't think you ever stop worrying about them. However, life happens and you deal with whatever it brings.
>
> I'll never forget the morning of June 25th. I got up, I had left my phone in the living room on the couch and couldn't hear it ring. I had several missed calls from Casey, and it was 5:30 in the morning. My heart was beating faster and faster as I returned the call. I prayed as I dialed, *please Lord, nothing bad.* She was at the hospital with Jeff in intensive care. He had a wreck. That's all I knew as I quickly got dressed and headed to San Antonio.
>
> The ensuing hours, days, weeks, and months were at best uncertain, as is life. The one certain thing, the one thing we can count on is God. God is a mystery. Perhaps the greatest mystery is how suffering and tragedy can bring a person into the presence of God in a state of worship, love and praise, but it does. It brought our family together also. Immediate family, in-laws, ex in-laws and family we barely knew. We are all much closer than before.
>
> I am so proud of Casey. She never lost her faith. She never doubted God. She never gave up on Jeff, or on God, to work miracles. He did work miracles, and the greatest is showing us he cares. This tragedy touched more lives than one can imagine, and it changed more also. One day we will all see God with our own eyes and our own bodies, and we will thank him for all the life changing experiences we have had. Thank you God for the miracle of bringing Jeff back and for bringing so many people closer to you.
>
> "Therefore encourage one other and build each other up, just as in fact you are doing" (1 Thessalonians 5:11).

The day after Jeff's birthday, he continued to make unexplainable progress. He was beginning to feed himself. He was able to hold the spoon and bring it to his mouth. A couple of times, he even scooped food from his plate on his own. Although he still couldn't remember names, he was recognizing more people.

During physical therapy, we were in the gym, and Jeff was throwing a ball; I saw him look over at an older gentleman. I watched Jeff's eyes and could see that mischievous twinkle in them. I suspected that he was going to throw the ball, but before I could do anything about it, there went the ball. He threw it right at that poor old guy. The guy was nice; he just laughed and threw the ball back. Jeff had a smile of satisfaction on his face.

Tremendous progress had already been made in the short time since Jeff woke up, but he continued to have this dazed look in his eyes. He was just oblivious to the reality of his situation. There was no concern for the future or the difficulties that he was having in the present. At this point, he seemed to be unburdened with the problems he was facing. When I looked at him, he would look back, but there was just this look of disorientation in his eyes. I could tell that he was not all there with me.

After three weeks of spending the majority of every single day at the hospital with Jeff, I finally went home for most of the day. I left in the morning and didn't go back to the hospital until the next day. It was really difficult to do, but I knew that I needed to take care of myself if I was going to take care of Jeff. I was starting to get very worn down and needed to get some real rest. I knew Jeff was safe with our families staying with him; he wasn't going to be alone. Again the phrase rings in my head, "It's a marathon, not a sprint." I needed to refresh myself to continue this journey.

Another notable accomplishment during this time was that Jeff was using the restroom. This was good news for him, and me. He no longer had to endure the pain of an in-and-out catheter every six hours, and I no longer had to hold him down while he had it done. It took a lot of time and patience. We had to try to take him to the restroom every two hours to ask him to go. Half the time, he didn't understand what was going on. The other half, he did, but didn't comprehend what was happening.

He would try to sit on the toilet with his pants on. When we would make him get up, he was baffled. Sometimes when I tried to pull his pants down, he would yank them back up, not understanding why I would do something like that. This process could take twenty minutes. If he didn't go, then we just had to try again later. But it was progress. We were moving forward.

Both of Jeff's sisters stayed with him that night. They told me that he told them he had to use the restroom, so they helped him get there. But when they got to the door, he turned around and said, "Wait here." It was the first time that he was aware of who was around him and what was appropriate or inappropriate to do around them.

> Journal update, Friday, July 15, 2011
>
> Today we had a family meeting with the doctors and therapists regarding Jeff's progress. On Tuesday, I wrote the update about praying for an impossible miracle; the doctors and therapists knew nothing about it. When they were talking about his progress, they said that at first everything was a lot of work, and it took forever to get Jeff to do anything, but they all said that on Wednesday, it was like a switch flipped, and all of a sudden, everything seemed easier, and he was catching on to everything much quicker. They couldn't explain it. I told them it was called prayer. So keep praying for the impossible miracle.

What else can I say but, "Praise the Lord!"? I asked for a miracle, and I was getting one. Jeff may not have been completely healed overnight, but he made such significant progress that it caught the attention of his therapists! If that's not a miracle in the making, I don't know what is. There is no way that can be a coincidence. They said, "It was like a switch flipped." Not only did a switch get flipped, but it happened the day that I prayed for Jeff's miracle. God flipped that switch for him. There were so many miracles that I was able to witness throughout this journey, but this one was the most obvious to me.

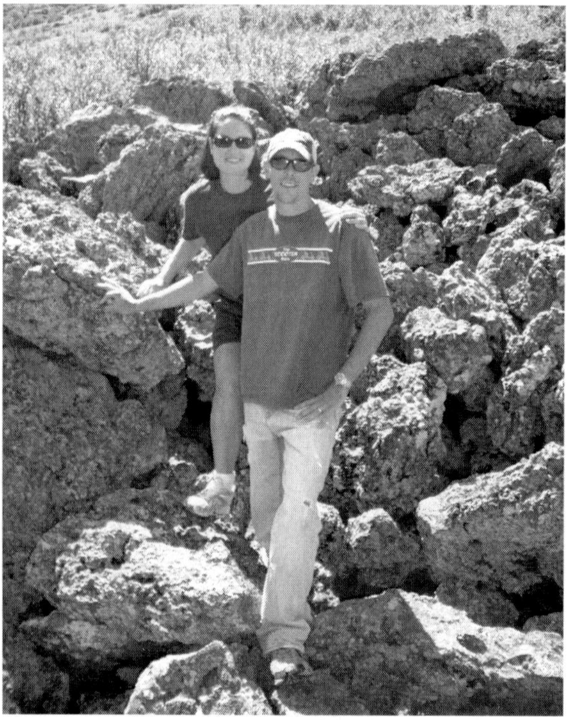

Before the accident, taken inside a volcano

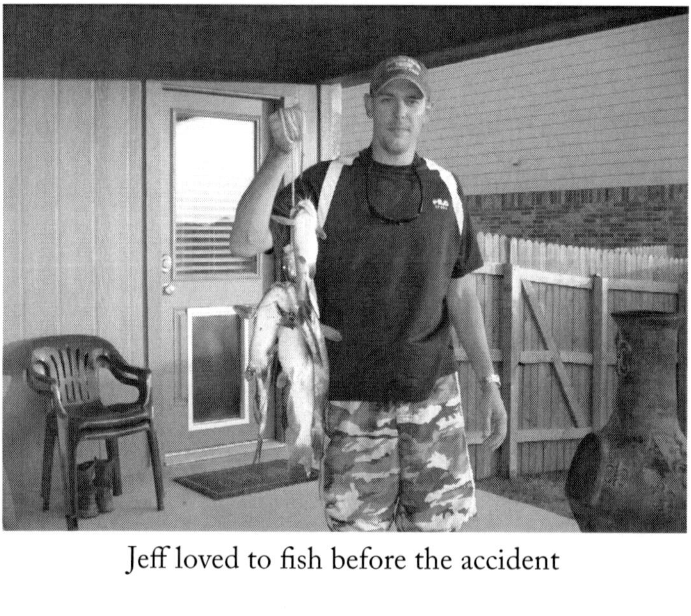

Jeff loved to fish before the accident

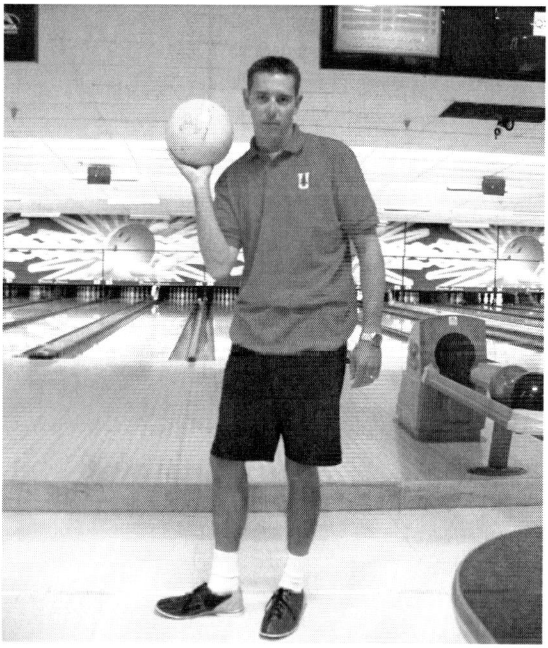

Bowling with friends

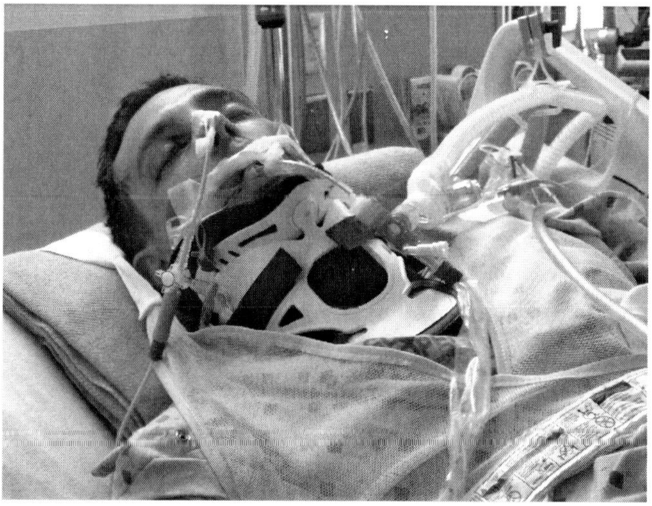

Day 2 after the accident

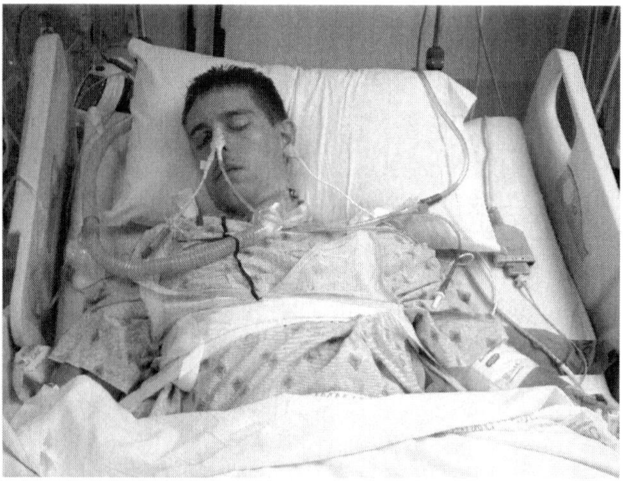

After the tracheotomy

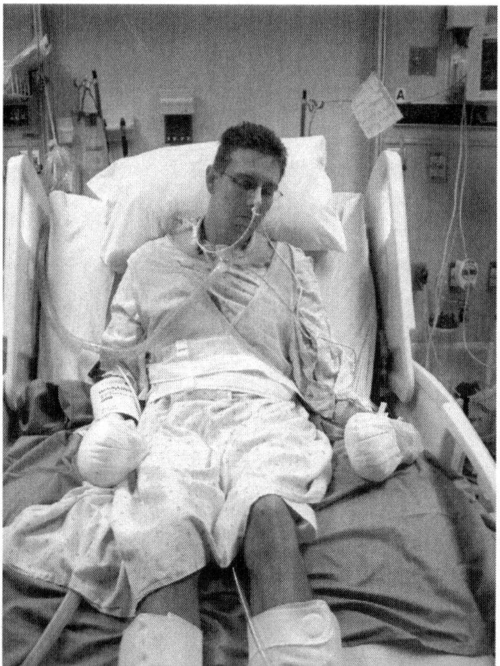

Day 9, putting Jeff in a sitting position

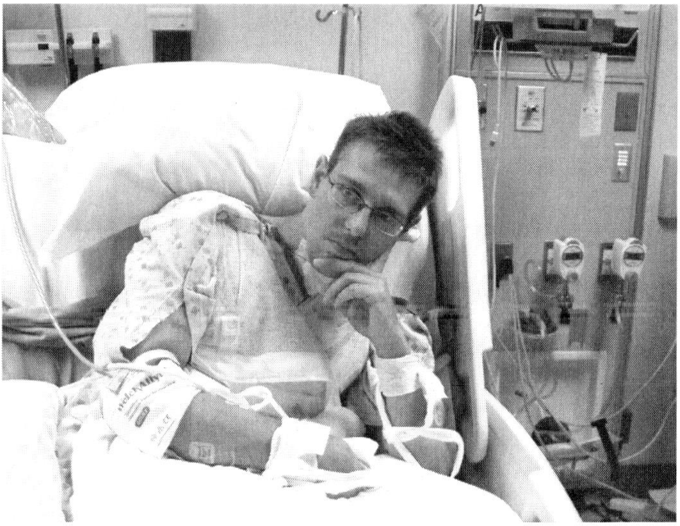

Day 10, some of the tubes have been removed
so Jeff is able to have his hands free

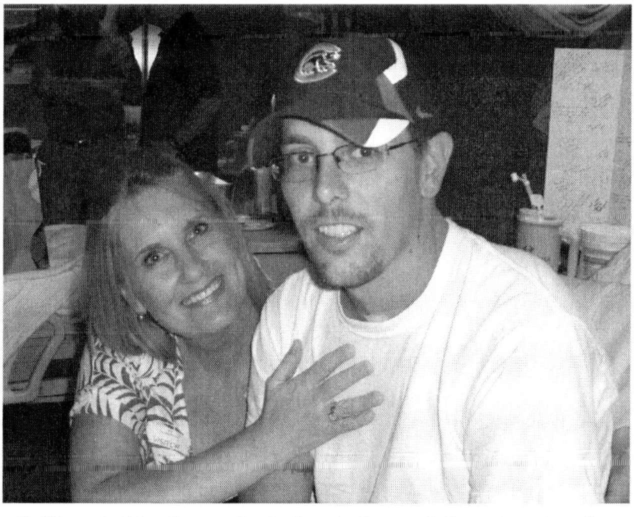

Jeff and Sheila at their birthday celebration in the
rehab hospital day 17 after the accident

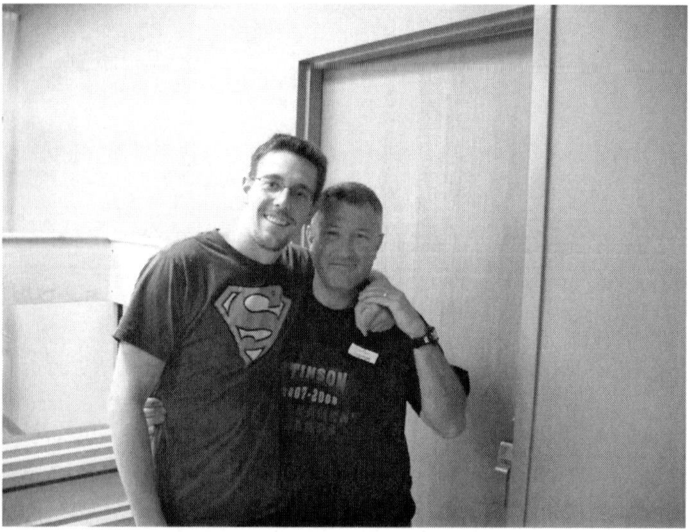

Jeff and his brother-in-law, about a month after the accident

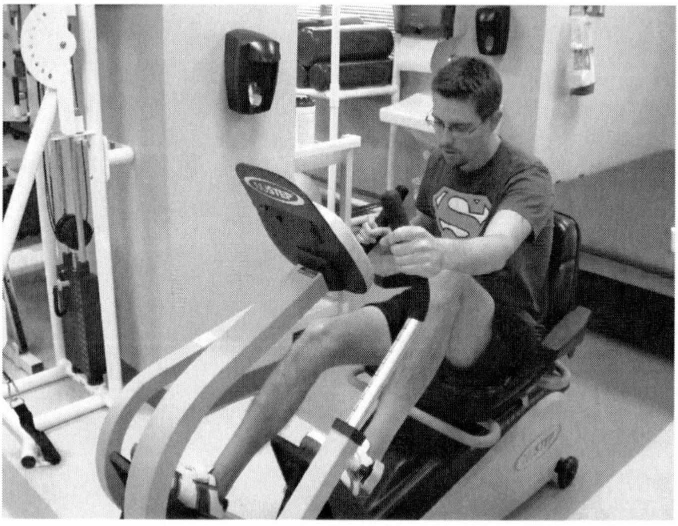

Doing some physical therapy

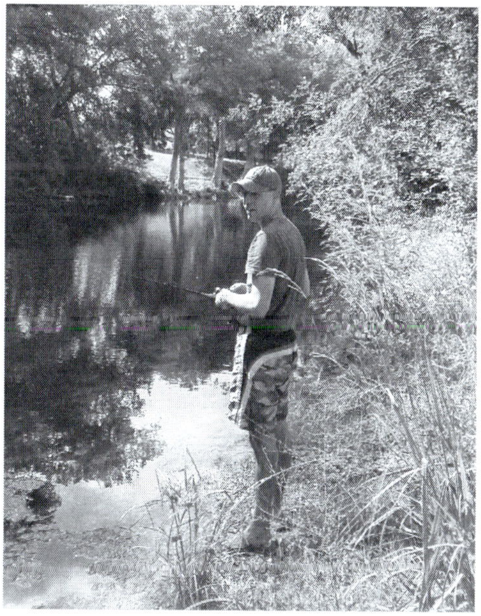

1st fishing trip after the accident

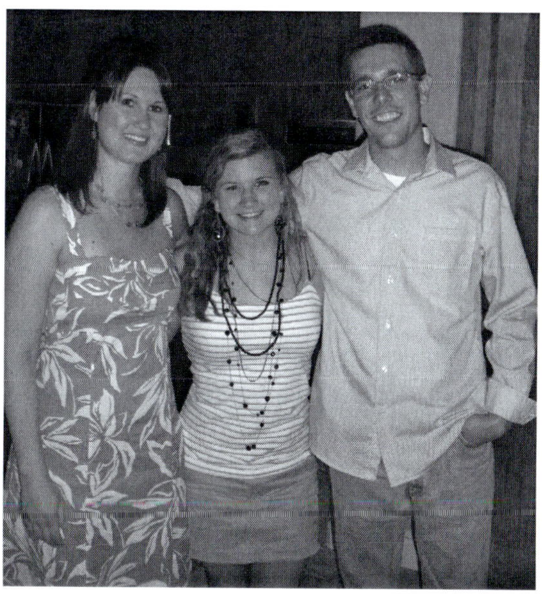

Jeff, Kelby, and I about 3 months after the accident

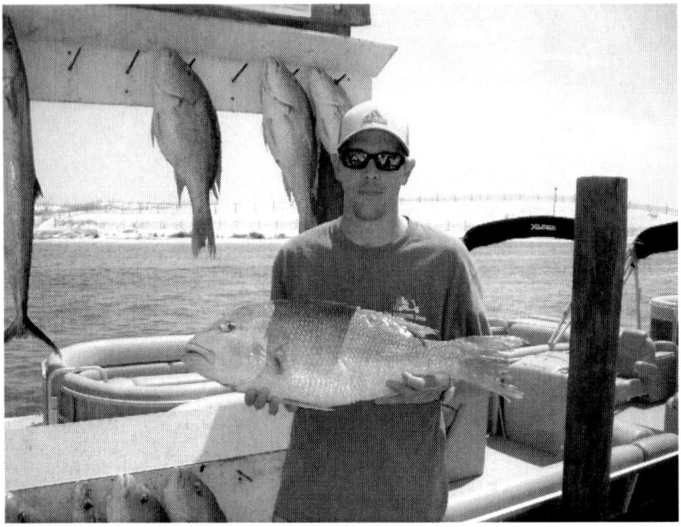

Deep sea fishing trip 1 year after the accident

FEARS AND STRUGGLES

Journal update, Monday, July 18, 2011

It was another busy day. The doctor wanted to wean Jeff from the bed he's in now, which is like an adult-size playpen, and into a regular hospital bed. That meant there was nothing to keep him from just getting up and walking out. It didn't go as well as we would have liked, and we are going to hold off on that for a while. On the brighter side, his walking has improved. In fact, a couple of times when he escaped into the hallway, he said, "See ya," and *ran* into another room. He did great in speech therapy today. He did several things he's never been able to do before. The therapist had Jeff repeat things she said, starting with sounds, then went to two-letter words, longer words, phrases, and sentences, and he was able to repeat everything she said! He was also able to finish opposite phrases. For example, she would say "up," and he would finish with "down," which he was never able to do before. So he is continuing to make progress.

I was talking to his physical therapist today, and she said it's great that he is making progress every day. I asked if that was normal. She told me that the quickness of his recovery is not normal; he is doing great. So again, thank you for the prayers, and keep them coming! Something specific I would like you to pray for is his impulsiveness. Right now, if he wants something, he just does it and

> doesn't think about the consequences, which could be dangerous for him. So pray that it gets better.

During this stage, I really struggled with my role as a wife. Reality was sinking in, and I was beginning to understand the truth that things were not going to be the same anymore. My future was going to be drastically different from anything that I had pictured. I wrestled with the fact that I wasn't sure if I had the patience or strength to take care of Jeff for the rest of my life. I knew that God had given me the strength to get this far, but how long would he carry me?

This stage of his recovery required a lot of patience. At first, I was doing really well with it. Just to get Jeff in or out of bed could take twenty to thirty minutes. His therapists told me several times that I was unbelievably patient with him. I tried to be patient with the process. I tried to be patient with Jeff. I knew that getting frustrated with Jeff and getting upset with him wouldn't help. He wouldn't understand why I was upset. So to me, it just made sense to be patient with him. I used every ounce of patience I had with Jeff. So when I was alone, I would break down.

I was frustrated with the process, irritated at the situation, discouraged that his recovery was going to take so long, and annoyed that it took so much energy to get Jeff to do the smallest of tasks, like getting out of bed or brushing his teeth. I was scared that they were going to send him home with me and that my patience would run out. But in front of Jeff, and everyone else, I was the rock.

However, it took its toll on me. For the first couple weeks that Jeff was in the acute rehab facility, I had a lot of tolerance. I knew that he didn't understand what we wanted him to do, so I was very calm and patient. But after a while, it got too vexing. He didn't understand why he wasn't able to do the things he wanted to do and would get aggressive.

He didn't grasp that he couldn't just walk around by himself because he could fall down. He couldn't comprehend that he couldn't just walk into other people's rooms. He didn't know his strength or that it wasn't all right to push or hit someone because that person was in his way. It was exhausting.

This specific day, he was being particularly difficult, and I just couldn't take it anymore. The doctor wanted to wean him from the Posey bed that he was in. She wanted him in a regular hospital bed. So during the day, I was supposed to leave the bed unzipped so he could get up as he pleased.

However, he was incredibly impulsive, constantly up and down and up and down. He wanted to go walk around in the halls or explore in his room, but it wasn't like he was able to do this by himself. I had to be next to him, holding on to him, to keep him from falling over. He didn't like that he couldn't be by himself. Getting away from me was his constant objective, often pushing me out of the way or trying to hit me. I was exhausted and just couldn't do it anymore.

"Jeff, where are you going? You can't leave the room without your socks and shoes," I reminded him. I had to repeat that every time he tried to walk out of the room. Sometimes, it was shoes; other times, it was his pants or a shirt. Sometimes, he would glare back at me and grudgingly put them on before bolting out the door again. But this time, he just kept going. He didn't care; he wanted to get out. The nurses had to stop him and help me get him back to the room to get his shoes on.

By about 5:00 p.m., I'd had enough. I couldn't control him or fight with him anymore. He had twisted my wrist when I tried to keep him from going in another patient's room. I finally had to get a couple of the nurses to help me get him back in his bed and zip him up. He was furious. He yelled a few choice words at me to let me know what he really thought.

"Let me out! I want out!" he shouted. When I wouldn't let him out, he began kicking and hitting the netting.

I was supposed to spend the night that night. I didn't know how I was going to keep up the energy I needed to continue doing this the rest of the day, let alone the rest of our lives. I had spent about twenty minutes trying to coax him back into his bed so I could sit down for a minute, and he just wouldn't go.

My aunt Sheila lived just down the road, so I finally had to call her to come and stay with him so I could go outside, sit in my car, and just cry. I had no idea how long he would be like this or if it would ever get better. How was I supposed to do this for the rest of my life? How could I take him home if he was going to be like that forever? I knew it wasn't him; I knew it was the injury, but that didn't make it easier. I was afraid to take him home because I was afraid that he would hurt me. I was afraid to be alone with my own husband.

About a year before Jeff's injury, I had attempted to train for a half marathon. I pushed myself, but when it got closer to the race, I got sick, then hurt my back, then was sick again. I was unable to train and gave up on running in the race. If I couldn't run a physical marathon, how was I going to run this metaphorical one? How was I going to keep up my strength and patience to do this for the rest of our lives?

I ended up going home that night. I spent a lot of time crying and praying. God made me realize that I didn't have to have the strength. I just had to trust in and lean on God. "Come to me, all you who are weary and burdened, and I will give you rest. Take my yoke upon you and learn from me, for I am gentle and humble in heart, and you will find rest for your souls. For my yoke is easy and my burden is light" (Matthew 11:28–30).

He sent his Holy Spirit to live in me, to be my strength, and to provide comfort. When I was at the end of my rope, I had to hand it over to Jesus. "Praise be to the God and Father of our Lord Jesus Christ, the Father of compassion and the God of all comfort, who comforts us in all our troubles, so that we can comfort those in any trouble with the comfort we ourselves receive from God" (2 Corinthians 1:3–4). God comforted me that night and gave me the strength I needed to continue the race. Now, I am able to use the troubles in my life to bring comfort to others as God brought comfort to me.

In less than a month from his accident, Jeff was roaming the halls regularly (with supervision) and was able to name some simple objects such as a sock, brush, scissors, etc. The fact that he could recognize and name specific objects was wonderful progress. He had terrible language aphasia. That is basically where Jeff might have a word in his head, but he would be unable to say it. Sometimes, he would say a different word; other times, he would make something up.

For example, if I held up a ball and asked him to name it, instead of saying ball, he might say sock, or he might say "bilgish." To him, it sounded right. He was unable to recognize, at this stage, that what was coming out of his mouth was not the same as what he thought was coming out. When we would tell him his answer was incorrect, he would seem puzzled. This would happen in his regular speech as well, causing a lot of frustration for him when we did not understand what he was trying to say. Being able to name even simple objects was a huge improvement and showed his continued development.

> We are thrilled to read of the progress Jeff is making and we continue to pray for his recovery, his safety as he explores, and for strength for each of you as you move through this together. We see God's hand in each entry! Hugs and Prayers...here if you need us for anything.
>
> —Bob and Melanie Linder

Just two days shy of the one month mark, the day had gone well. I was still able to see Jeff's continued improvement and recognize the miracles that were continuing to unfold. But, when I got home that evening, it was as if I finally hit a wall. I had been so strong up to this point. If I started crying, I was able to stop when I wanted to. I was being the rock for Jeff. Even previously, that night in the bathtub when I was bawling and screaming at God, I was able to turn off the tears when I was done. This night, I couldn't.

Throughout the day, things just kept piling up, and my stress level reached an all-time high. With my focus primarily on mine and Jeff's journey, it was easy to forget that others were dealing with their pain in their own way. They couldn't comprehend what I was going through any more than I could comprehend what they were going through. No one intentionally set out to hurt the other, but at times, it was inevitable. Looking back, I know I overreacted, but my emotions got the best of me.

Earlier that night, I received a phone call from a friend. She informed me that someone was starting rumors about Jeff and how his accident "really" happened. I didn't understand how someone could be so cruel. How could they see the pain that we were going through and then try to make it worse? Not to mention it wasn't even true; but that didn't stop people from believing it.

Shortly after that unpleasant conversation, I got a call from Jeff's sister. She wasn't happy about my "picture of the day." I had started an online picture journal where I took a picture every day for a year. Today's picture was of Jeff, in a helmet, walking up some steps to mark another milestone. His sister, most likely concerned about Jeff's self-esteem, asked me to take the picture down. At the time I thought, *If I want to post a picture of my husband to share his progress and receive encouragement from friends, what right did she have to take that from me?* Looking back now, I know she didn't mean to upset me; she was just trying to protect her brother. But I couldn't see that at the time. So in my anger, I drew a picture of a sad face on a piece of paper and posted that instead.

That phone call was the last straw. I had dealt with enough. I couldn't hold it together anymore. I started crying and couldn't stop. I didn't know what to do. I cried for hours. I wanted someone to come over and hold me while I cried, but it was late, and I didn't want to make anyone drive over to my house. People had helped me so much; I didn't want to be more of a burden, and I knew it hurt my family to see me in pain.

I finally called my best friend. After erroneously accusing her of being the cause of the rumor, she just listened to me through my sobs. She told me that she was surprised this meltdown hadn't happened sooner. She told me I was stubborn and that I just needed to let go and give everything to God. While God was providing me with strength, I was still trying to find it on my own. The tears would not subside, and eventually I cried myself to sleep.

The next day my dad was preaching at his church, so Jeff's entire family was there. I sat in the pew behind them and didn't say a word before or after the service. I was still upset but knew that it was not the time or place to say anything. Of course, in my dad's sermon, he talked about forgiveness and letting go of problems that are out of your control. *Gee, thanks, Dad. I couldn't wallow in my self-pity a little longer?* (He had no idea what I had gone through the previous night, but God did, and he used my dad's sermon to talk to me). No more wallowing; it was time to forgive and move on. I had bigger problems that I needed to worry about, and my focus needed to return to Jeff and his recovery.

TRANSITIONS

> We are honored to call your name before our Lord. Keep God's Word before you every day throughout the day… it will be your peace and strength. Blessings to you as you make the transition today.
>
> —Steve and Celia Peace

Many people react negatively to change. Life would be so much easier if things would stay the same. For a person with a brain injury, this is especially true. Jeff thrived on routine and predictability. When something changed, he tended to take a few steps back. Sometimes it could be steps in his progress, other times it would be steps in his behavior. However, just as in life, change is inevitable when dealing with a brain injury. Sometimes he did great, other times it was more difficult.

Day 31 was a big day. It was nearing the end of Jeff's stay at the first rehab facility, so a day pass was granted to test how Jeff would do in a car. He did much better than expected. Other than keeping his seatbelt on, we didn't have any problems.

The first stop was to go through a drive-thru to pick up lunch. Then we went to my aunt's house to eat and hang out for a while since she only lived a few minutes down the road from the rehab facility. He enjoyed interacting with people outside the hospital.

When we returned to the hospital however, Jeff became very agitated. He didn't understand why he had to go back. The hospital was making him stir crazy and he wanted to leave! Expressing himself was still difficult so Jeff let us know he was upset by throwing things on the floor, and pouting like a child. I felt so bad, but I knew this was the best thing for him.

As we were getting closer to Jeff possibly coming home, I had a lot of questions for the doctors. One of the concerns I had was very personal but caused me a lot of anxiety. I share this because I know that there are spouses out there with the same questions but are too afraid or embarrassed to ask. I wanted to know how, if, or when to interact with my husband intimately.

I had many fears surrounding this. I knew that sex was not anywhere in the near future; Jeff was more like my child than my husband at that stage, but I wanted to know when or if it would be alright in the future. I finally just decided to face the awkwardness and talk to Jeff's doctor about it. Without going into too much detail, I can say that the doctor answered my questions delicately and professionally, and put my mind at ease.

While I was deeply concerned about these very personal issues, other people were not quite as respectful of its personal nature. One friend, who I'm sure was only trying to be helpful, tried to give me some advice. She informed me that she had read a study about people with brain injuries. Apparently, sex is good for the brain and can aid in the healing process. So jokingly she told me that we should be having lots of sex to help him get better.

I laughed with her, but on the inside, I was crying. First of all, we were in a hospital with no locks on the door and zero privacy. Second, I was literally taking care of Jeff and raising him as if he were my child. It didn't feel right thinking about having sex with him. The doctor had advised that it wasn't good to be entertaining those thoughts at that time. Not to mention the fact that more often than not, Jeff was mean and aggressive toward me, and the last thing I wanted to do was be intimate with him.

In the meantime, the acute rehab facility was no longer able to meet Jeff's needs, and he was about to be discharged. However, we were again blessed to find a more long-term facility that would accept Jeff for a few weeks. This was much better than trying to take Jeff home in the state he was in.

This is just another testimony of how God worked miracles for us. Every time I was concerned about what would happen next, God took care of it. He calmed my fears of having Jeff home too soon. He not only provided a place for Jeff to go next, but he also provided financially for him to go there. Jeff had not been at his job long enough to have health insurance and, obviously, was not getting any more paychecks in the near future. I wasn't going to be able to return to school at the beginning of the school year and take care of Jeff full-time, so I ended up quitting my job. We had an income of zero and no immediate solutions on the horizon. But that didn't matter to God; he is bigger than our financial problems.

Before Jeff was able to move to the new facility, he needed to be able to stay in a regular hospital bed instead of the Posey. To get him ready for that, we had to start letting him sleep in one. It was incredibly nerve-racking. When I stayed the night with him, I hardly slept at all. I was afraid that he was going to get up and set off the alarm. Yet, if I turned the alarm off, he could get up in the middle of the night and wander out into the hallway without being noticed. If the nurses were in another patient's room or away from the nurses' station, he could easily get in the elevator and go downstairs or walk to the stairwell himself. He was not sturdy enough to walk up and down the stairs without falling so that posed a major threat.

I would try to explain to him that once we turned the bed alarm on, he had to tell me before getting up so I could turn it back off. Otherwise, the alarm would sound. But he wasn't able to remember; he would get up to go to the restroom and set off the alarm. That was one heck of a way to wake up! I would jump out of my bed to see what was going on, and he would just be standing by his bed, looking at it quizzically, wondering why it was screaming at him.

I had good reason to be afraid too. The next day, Jeff gave me a huge scare. I was walking around the hallway with him, and he decided he wanted to go down the stairs. He opened the door to the stairwell and went in. He had walked up and down a couple of steps with his therapist, but he was not ready to go down an entire flight of stairs; he was still too unbalanced. I followed him in, trying to get him back in the hallway, but he went straight for the stairs. I let go of the door to block him, and it locked from the other side. So there I was, locked in the stairwell with Jeff trying to push me out of the way to go down. I started banging on the door while still trying to keep him from taking the first step down the stairs. I was afraid that he would fall, but I also feared that he would push me down the stairs if I was in his way. A nurse finally heard me banging and screaming and came to help. I took him back to the room after that so I could catch my breath. My heart was pounding!

During this time, Jeff had to take a lot of medications but was unable to swallow pills whole. Most of them we were able to crush up and mix into yogurt to give them to him. However, he also had to take fish oil. This was not a crushable pill and was way too big for him to try to swallow. We had to puncture the capsule, pour out the fish oil, and then mix it into his yogurt. Not only did this not taste good, but it smelled like rotten fish!

He had gotten to the stage where he could feed himself, so I was trying to let him feed himself his fish oil yogurt. Apparently, he thought it looked like lotion and rubbed it into his hands! It smelled awful for days!

Then, I didn't learn my lesson, and the next day I was trying to get him to take the fish oil yogurt. I held the cup out in my hand with a spoon, but he picked up the cup. I was afraid he was going to rub it on his hands again, so I asked him to give it to me. Maybe I should have been a little more specific because he poured it in my hand. So we got to smell like fish together. For days, every time I brought my hands to my face, I could smell it. Needless to say, I was very glad when he was able to swallow that pill!

After 5 weeks, Jeff moved to his 2nd rehab facility. My brother had stayed with Jeff the night before his move and said Jeff didn't sleep at all. I guess he understood that he was moving somewhere and was anxious about it. Jeff's healing brain needed a lot of sleep, and not getting any made him very grumpy the next day. The transition from the hospital to the first rehab facility was in an ambulance, so I didn't have to worry about Jeff's safety. This time however, we were not afforded that luxury.

I rode in the backseat with Jeff while my dad drove us the 30 minutes to the new hospital. Child-locks were used on the back doors for fear Jeff would decide he didn't want to be in the car anymore while we were driving down the highway. Thankfully, that didn't happen, and we all made it in one piece.

While he didn't try to escape, Jeff was not happy about being in the car for such a long time. He kept unbuckling his seatbelt and squirming all over the backseat. The entire ride, he was agitated. Once we arrived, Jeff was much happier. The new scenery provided a distraction, and he was happy to be out of the car.

The doctors warned us that moving Jeff to a new place could cause him to take a few steps back or cause some problems. Patients with brain injuries do not like change. They were right. He was glad to be out of the first hospital, but very upset that he was moved to another one. For a few days after the move, he was very agitated and not in a place mentally that he could understand why being at home wasn't an option.

It was explained to me that people with a brain injury remember themselves the way they were at their best. So Jeff didn't think of himself as having a brain injury; he remembered himself before the accident. He didn't understand why we wouldn't let him go home. Until Jeff was able to comprehend that there was something wrong with him, it made keeping him in a hospital a constant source of frustration.

It was very trying on me. When I say that Jeff was agitated, I don't mean that he complained a lot. He could be violent. He would throw things at me, say very hurtful things, push me out of the way, or try to hit me. This particular day, he was acting so bad that the nurses had to come in and calm him down. He wasn't cooperating with his therapists, and then when he was eating lunch, he began throwing food and silverware at me.

Jeff is not a mean person. Before the accident, if he got upset at me, it was because I did something to really deserve it, and he never got physical with me. So this was a very different side of him. The worst part about it was that he would be nice to other people, and then as soon as they would leave the room, he was right back to being cruel to me. The doctors told me that it was a backhanded compliment. He felt like he could trust me and was comfortable with me, so I was the one he took everything out on. I always tried to remember that it wasn't him; it was the brain injury, but it was very difficult not to take it personally.

Here was this man that I loved. I had just spent eight days at his bedside, wondering if he was ever going to wake up. I had spent the past month looking after and taking care of him. I had given him every ounce of energy and patience that was in me. Yet he was no longer the person that I married. Instead of the sweet, thoughtful, loving, and gentle man that I married, Jeff had been replaced with this mean, angry, hurtful, and uncaring person whom I didn't know. I had no way of knowing if this was a phase that he would eventually grow out of or if he was going to be like that for the rest of our lives.

Journal update, Wednesday, August 3, 2011

Jeff seems to be settling in better now. He was less agitated yesterday than on Monday. He has a very busy schedule. He still gets three hours of therapy each day. However, like I said before, it is a little more challenging for him, which is good. He also meets with a psychologist for about thirty minutes each day. Then, he works with a lady in the transitional living program, where he works on things to help him be more independent, such as cooking, as well as social skills. Today, he is supposed to cook a meal and watch a movie. We will see how that goes. Once he gets more situated, they hope to be able to take him on outings to get him used to being in the community again and learning how to interact with people in a different environment.

He still continues to make progress. He seems to be more aware of his surroundings, and some memory is starting to come back. He is sometimes even able to tell you that he is in the hospital because he got in a wreck. I don't think he actually remembers that, but he is remembering us telling him he was in an accident. He hasn't been able to say he was on a four-wheeler, but he understands it was some kind of wreck.

Specific prayer requests for now are that he continues to make speedy progress, especially right now. He will only be at this facility for two weeks, so it is important he makes as much progress as possible because we don't know where he will be after this and if he will have to come home or not. Also, pray that we are able to get him into another facility after this.

I also want to thank everyone again for all the prayers, love, and support. I know I keep saying it, but I really cannot thank you enough. I have been overwhelmed by the love of friends and family. Thank you to everyone who has brought meals, cleaned my house, done laundry, walked dogs, come for visits, prayed, been a listening ear, donated

> money, written in the guest book, sent cards, and so many other things. I know everyone keeps saying that I'm strong, but it is only by the power of God and your loving support. So thank you, thank you, thank you.

"God Will meet all your needs according to the riches of his glory in Christ Jesus" (Philippians 4:19). More than anyone else on earth, God knew and understood what I needed. He created me. He knew every detail of my life that needed to be taken care of, from walking my dogs to giving me encouraging words to help me through difficult days. No matter what my need was, God sent someone to help with it or provided the help himself through comfort, strength, or peace. "You have searched me Lord, and you know me. You know when I sit and when I rise, you perceive my thoughts from afar" (Psalm 139:1–2). When people could only see how I was doing from the outside, God was searching my heart. He saw every minute detail of my life and identified what I needed at that moment.

UPS AND DOWNS

I started reading different books about brain injuries; many of them discussed the toll that it can take on families. Many statistics regarding marriages after a spouse has a brain injury show that 40–50 percent (and some professionals say it is higher) end in divorce. The caregivers end up feeling isolated and trapped. Wives found their spouses "selfish, childish, demanding, and dependent."[6]

This was not an option for me. I took my vows of marriage seriously, and I was not going to leave Jeff. I'm in no way judging others who couldn't make their marriage work, and I completely understand why a spouse would leave in this situation. I understand that in some circumstances involving brain injuries, divorce happens to keep the uninjured spouse from becoming injured.

In fact, someone was trying to comfort me and said that I was being a supportive wife by sharing a story of another wife she knew that didn't stick by her husband. She said that the husband suffered a brain injury, and the wife couldn't handle the difficulties, so she divorced him. However, later the husband recovered and remarried someone else.

I defended that wife. The woman telling me the story made a comment that if the wife had just stuck around, things would have gotten better. She had no idea what it is like for the spouse of someone with a brain injury. While that husband may have recovered, he would never be the same man that he was when his wife married him. He may have seemed fine from an outsider's view, but to the woman that had to live with him every day, there were difficulties that couldn't be seen by others. His new wife didn't know what he was like before his injury and thus wasn't disappointed when he wasn't the same.

I understand that. I completely sympathize with that wife. Jeff may seem fine to those that don't spend every day with him. To me though, there are small differences that may never go away. Little things that didn't use to bother him can easily upset him now. There is a dependency that did not exist before the accident. Small decisions that he should be able to make now require my advice. He is more sensitive to everything and can be easily brought down. Remembering simple directions can become problematic, so asking him to run errands is almost impossible. I have to go with him to the store because he can't remember which bag of dog food to buy. Now, rarely wanting to go to group gatherings, Jeff is no longer the social guy that he used to be. He has to be dragged to most functions now. These may seem like minor details, but if you were married to a spouse who was the "head of the household" and always made the decisions, it could cause some serious problems.

However, I also feel that our society has placed more value on the individual finding happiness than in couples making a marriage last. If a spouse is making the other miserable, it is socially acceptable to leave. I had to figure out a way to make it work. And I knew that I could not turn to just anyone to find that help. I needed to take advice only from those who valued marriage the way that I did.

Still, I was terrified; I didn't want to be married to an abusive spouse or even one that just yelled at me all the time. I have never had a lot of patience. When Jeff and I argued before, I was always the one to lose my temper. Gary Thomas argues in *Sacred Marriage* that

> If the purpose of marriage was simply to enjoy an infatuation and make me "happy," then I'd have to get a "new"

> marriage every two or three years. But if I really want to see God transform me from the inside out, I'd need to concentrate on changing *myself* rather than on changing my *spouse*...If I'm married only for happiness, and my happiness wanes for whatever reason, one little spark will burn the entire forest of my relationship. But if my aim is to proclaim and model God's ministry of reconciliation, my endurance will be fireproof.[7]

When Jeff and I got married, I not only said vows to Jeff, but I said them to God. Marriage is not just a relationship between the two of us; it is a union with God as well. My focus had to be higher than just my relationship with my husband. It had to be based on my relationship with God. I knew that I had to change. I could not be the wife that existed before if I was going to make our marriage work. I had to learn how to express myself without losing my temper, how to have patience. Every time I lost my temper before, there was always this little voice in the back of my mind telling me that I had another choice, but I always ignored it. I couldn't ignore it anymore. I had to listen and keep my calm if I wanted to stay married. I made the choice to become a better wife, and in turn, I learned how to respond to Jeff and how to stay calm. I didn't just push all my feelings down; I found people that I trusted whom I was able to talk to. I worked my feelings out in healthy ways instead of splattering them all over Jeff.

I spent some time in prayer about it, and I confided in a good friend whom I knew also did not see divorce as an option in her marriage. I knew that if I tried to talk to someone that did not have the same convictions about marriage as me, I would end up being counseled to divorce. Most people suggest divorce when circumstances seem impossible. I did not even want to hear that divorce was an option. I didn't want anyone to tell me that it would be all right if I left. God granted me supernatural wisdom and patience in our situation. Eventually, when I didn't lose my patience, I stood firm with Jeff and let him know what was and was not acceptable, his aggression subsided. It was not overnight, but little by little, it got better.

At this hospital, I was invited to join a support group of other wives that also had husbands with brain injuries. This was one of the most helpful resources that I discovered in this entire journey. I wish I had found it sooner. I was finally able to talk to other wives and ask what they were doing to cope. I was able to learn that what I was feeling and going through was normal. I wasn't a horrible person for thinking some of the things I did. They were thinking the same things! They were asking the same questions! They cried with me and laughed with me. They encouraged me when Jeff wasn't doing so well and rejoiced with me when he made progress. In turn, I was able to share with them what I was doing to cope. If you have a spouse with a brain injury, or any type of life-changing matter, I highly suggest that you find a support group.

On the other hand, it also made reality sink in for me just a little more. The two wives that I connected with had husbands that had brain injuries about four months prior to Jeff's. It gave me a glimpse into what my future was going to look like. They were both still dealing with aggression in their spouses.

"I feel like the evil witch sometimes," Stacy said. "When we are at home, Curtis will yell at me for no reason. I walk on egg-shells around him, trying not to do anything that would upset him. There is always something though. He is very rarely nice to me. Then we go out in public, or to see the doctor, and he is as nice as can be. I'm afraid people think I'm making it up because he's like a different person around me than he is around other people."

"I know you aren't making it up, Jeremy does the same thing to me," Victoria confirmed.

I knew what they were both talking about. Just in rehab, Jeff was already beginning to do the same thing around me. His demeanor could change immediately if someone walked in the room and he was being mean to me. How long was this going to last? These wives were still struggling with it.

Up to this point, Jeff wasn't able to do anything by himself; he had to have supervision twenty-four seven. Even supervised, he would try to go out the fire escape doors. I was with him one time when he went out one of the doors. He was frustrated and wanted to leave the hospital. I explained he couldn't go out the fire exit door, or the alarm would sound, but he did it anyway. A security guard had to come and check things out and had to talk to him about not using the door. Another time, my aunt and cousins were staying with him. They were walking around the halls, and he walked right out the door. When the alarm sounded, he looked at Aunt Sheila, pointed his finger at her, and said, "Why weren't *you* watching me?"

It was a big deal when he was able to see the No Exit sign on the door and know that he wasn't supposed to go out that door. It made me very nervous letting him walk around the halls by himself. I was worried he would wander into someone else's room or figure out how to get out of the locked unit. Nevertheless, it was time to let go and allow him to explore and learn on his own. It was important for his development to make mistakes. It was very much like raising a child.

Since Jeff was recognizing signs, the doctors wanted us to give him more freedom, so he was walking around the hallways of the brain injury unit by himself. As long as Jeff didn't say anything, he looked normal. He didn't have any broken bones, and all his scrapes and bruises had healed by this time. If you didn't know him, he didn't look like a patient. So he discovered that if he stood by the locked door, someone would eventually come through, and he could get out. Since he didn't look like a patient, no one questioned it.

After that, the nurses posted big red signs on all the doors for Jeff that told him to stop. While it scared me that Jeff was able to get out of the locked unit, the signs seemed to work. This was another great accomplishment. He was able to read a sign and understand what it meant. He knew he wasn't supposed to go through the door if it had the red sign up. It was also huge that he had figured out which doors went outside the unit as opposed to another patient's room and that he was able to do problem solving on how to get out of the doors.

Jeff loved to barbecue before his accident. He was really good at it too. On August 10th, day 46, Jeff got to barbecue at the rehab facility as part of the transitional living program. He made us some hamburgers. I tried my hardest not to tell him how to do it. The burgers were only about halfway done when he put the cheese on them. Then he flipped them after he had already put the cheese on top. He was also trying to cook them over the part of the pit that didn't have the flame. The meat was a little rare, and the buns a little burnt, but he did it by himself! He seemed proud of himself when he was done which made me happy.

We also got the good news this day that the rehab hospital would be able to lengthen Jeff's stay by another week at no cost to us! This was great news because Jeff was still too impulsive, confused, and agitated to go home. I wouldn't have been able to handle him on my own.

On top of him being too impulsive, for whatever reason, Jeff did not like doing anything with me. He didn't want to play games, work on therapy, or have a conversation with me, nothing. He either wanted to walk around or just sit on his bed and do nothing. Both of which he got bored with very quickly, so we alternated between them a lot. He would never sit still long enough for me to read a book or do anything on my own. I couldn't play games on my phone because he would get mad that he didn't have his phone. When he walked around, he just got frustrated that he couldn't leave the hospital. He would ask me to walk around with him but then get upset that I was by his side constantly. If I left him alone, he often got lost, then would be angry with me for leaving him alone. No matter what I did, I wasn't able to satisfy him.

I stayed the night with him one evening, and he found some popcorn. He wanted to eat it but was convinced that the bathroom sink was the microwave. When I wouldn't let him pop the popcorn in the sink, he threw a fit and threw it away. Then he threw his shoes and glasses across the room and crawled in bed. I knew he wasn't really mad at me, so I crawled in the bed with him and scratched his back. After a while, he apologized. Then he fell asleep while I scratched his back.

I don't know why he wouldn't do anything with me. My assumption is that he associated me with keeping him in the hospital. Since I was the one that spent the most time with him, I was constantly telling him no. No, he couldn't go out to his truck. No, he couldn't leave the hospital. No, he couldn't go home. Even though everyone else said the same thing, I said it the most. So I guess he was just frustrated with me and didn't want to do anything with me. However, when I was gone, he would call me constantly and ask what I was doing and when I was coming back. He didn't want me there, but he didn't want me gone either. It was impossible to keep him happy.

Apparently, our brains don't like it when there are gaps in our memory. Jeff's brain had a lot of gaps in his memory that he wasn't able to fill. So instead of just having gaps, the brain fills them in with made-up memories; they are called confabulations. When the brain does this, it creates a memory that didn't happen, and the person believes it's true.

Jeff did this a lot. Sometimes it was small things that sounded believable, like he had tacos for breakfast instead of the eggs and bacon that he really had. Other times, they were very elaborate and may or may not sound believable. It didn't matter how unreal the story sounded; to Jeff, it was the truth.

Sometimes, the confabulations were just funny. One Sunday, I was at church and called Jeff in between church and Sunday school. His brother-in-law was staying with him. When I asked what he was doing, he told me that they had just gone fishing, and now they were sitting in the church parking lot, playing the banjo.

Other times, they caused problems. Before his accident, Jeff had a Dodge truck that he loved. I had to sell it since we were no longer able to make the payments. Many of his confabulations had to do with his truck. Convinced that his truck was out in the parking lot, he constantly wanted to go out and get something from it. Other times, he wanted me to take the truck somewhere so it was safe because he wasn't able to drive it. When I would try to tell him that his truck wasn't in the parking lot, he would get so cross with me. He always wanted to go out to see it, but he wasn't allowed to leave the hospital. One day, he was convinced that we had left the hospital the day before and didn't understand why we weren't able to leave again. He thought I was lying to him, which just caused him to be even more irritated with me.

Then, after 48 days, Jeff was finally having some windows of clarity. He actually remembered that he had been mean to me, and then apologized for it. He would even tell me he wasn't sure why he was like that. The doctor says that those windows will come in stages, and there will be good and bad days.

You have no idea how surprised and excited I was to hear Jeff apologize to me for being mean. For one thing, he actually realized that what he had done was wrong. It was the first sign that he was able to determine right from wrong. Then he *remembered* that he had done something wrong. He was starting to form real memories, not just confabulations! Finally, he was able to know to make amends for what he remembered he had done wrong.

This was such a sweet moment. We were lying on his bed together, watching TV. I looked over at him, and he appeared to be thinking really hard.

"What are you thinking about?" I asked.

"I'm sorry for being mean to you," he answered. It took him awhile to find the right words to get the sentence out, but he said it. We had a great conversation about what he had done, that he felt bad about it, and that he didn't understand why he would act like that. He told me that he didn't have a reason for being mean; he just did it. I finally felt like I was talking to *my* husband again for the first time since his accident. It only lasted a couple minutes, but I had a glimpse into what he could be again. I finally had hope that the man that I married might come back.

Learning Independence

> I am at a loss for words, your faith, your strength and a never dying love for the man you married. I know your continued support of Jeff through the bad and the good has helped him reach the unreachable......May God continue to give you and Jeff the strength to reach the top of that mountain. You are BOTH going to do it!!! My prayers will continue for you both. Much love to you and Jeff!
>
> —Pat Hermes

I might have mentioned it before, but I like to be in control. With Jeff having the mental capacity of a five-year-old, I had become very motherly and protective of him. I had a hard time letting him do anything by himself because I didn't want him to do it incorrectly. He needed to learn how to do things on his own, without me constantly telling him how it should be done. On the other hand, I had to learn how to let go and give him the space he needed to learn those skills.

Sunday, August 14th, was a very difficult day for me. Until now, Jeff had consistently only been mean to me but nice to everyone else. But on this particular day, Jeff's family was staying with him, while I was at church. Jeff began to get mean and told them to leave and that he didn't want anyone around. So they called me, told me that he wanted to be alone, and they left. It was the first time since he was unconscious in the ICU that he had been without friends or family.

I was angry and scared. I knew that we needed to start letting him be on his own a little, but not quite like that. I wanted to explain to Jeff that we were leaving to give him some independence, not leave because he threw a fit. I had been there and seen him throw fits. He kicked me out of the room numerous times, but I didn't leave the hospital. I went and sat in the waiting room until he cooled off, and then he wanted me back in there with him. The way I saw it, Jeff threw a fit, and his family thought it would be best to leave him, not realizing that he was probably going to forget about it in ten minutes and wonder where everyone was and why he was alone in the hospital.

I got there as soon as I could and let Jeff know I was there. He did want to be alone, so I sat in the waiting room. I sat there all afternoon. I would go in to check on him and let him know that I was still there. I sat there for six hours until my aunt got there to spend the night. I guess it really was time to give him some freedom. For someone who likes to be alone, he hadn't had a moment to himself for seven weeks.

I really struggled with giving Jeff independence. I was afraid he was going to hurt himself again. People kept telling me that I needed to let go and let him figure things out on his own, but I was afraid. I had never raised a child or witnessed the developmental stages they go through. I was terrified that he would do something that could potentially cause himself more harm. It was like a mother of a five-year-old going from playing with keys to driving a car. I didn't know how to do it, and I didn't want to be forced. I needed to let go at my own pace. Yes, I needed nudging and advice, but I wanted to be the one to make the decision; I didn't want to be forced.

I remember venting to my dad about it one day. "They just don't understand, Dad! They've already experienced letting him go in gradual stages. I don't get to! They want me to just completely let go, and I can't!"

"Casey, I understand how you feel," he replied. "I felt the same way when you moved out. You probably don't know this, but the day you left, I sat on the couch and cried. I know you had already lived on your own once before, but I didn't want to see you get hurt again. I knew it was time to let you go. You had to learn to make your own mistakes."

Ouch! You mean I wasn't the only one that had ever experienced these feelings? My dad helped me realize that even though this situation was different, I was not the only one to ever experience this emotional pain. It was time to let go. It was time to let Jeff make his own mistakes.

The next day, Jeff was a completely different person. He was sweet and affectionate towards me—constantly wanting to hold me, and apologizing for being mean. I was even able to talk to him about what happened and why he was in the hospital. Since he was doing so well and wanted to be on his own, we decided that we would let him spend the night at the hospital by himself.

This night was one of the most difficult nights I had since Jeff started waking up. The nurses were confident that he would be safe enough not to have someone in the room with him and assured me that they would keep an eye out in case he came into the hallway.

He would get confused a lot and was unable to find the restroom. He would wander out into the hallway and into other people's rooms, looking for it. He would also get up really early in the morning (sometimes 4:00 or 5:00 a.m.) and want to take a shower. However, he wouldn't be able to find an item of clothing that he needed, so he would throw his clothes all over the room and start throwing things in the trash. It was also possible that he could wander out of the locked unit since he had already figured out how to get out, or he could escape out the emergency exit. I was concerned one of these things might happen.

Then to make matters worse, Jeff told me that he didn't want me to leave. After all the times he wanted me to go, now that I was finally ready, he wasn't. I explained to him what we were doing and that he was going to be alone in the room for the night, but promised I would be back first thing in the morning. He begged me not to go. He told me that I was leaving him. In my head, I was thinking that once he came home, I would be there with him anyway, so why did he have to be alone in the hospital? But I knew that we needed to give him more independence. He needed to figure out how to ask the nurses for help if he needed something. He had to figure out how to do things without someone standing next to him telling him. I knew that if I stayed, he was never going to learn to do anything for himself because I would always be there to tell him how to do it correctly. He needed to make mistakes; he needed to learn for himself, and I needed to learn how to start letting go.

He practiced calling me and the nurses, and I assured him over and over that I was staying with his parents and would just be a few miles away. I told him that he could call me if he needed anything, that I could be there within a matter of minutes, and that I would be back first thing in the morning. I cried the whole way over to his parents' house, where I was greeted with open arms by his mom.

"He's going to be fine," she assured me.

"He didn't just tell you that you left him!" I unfairly snapped back. I'm sure she wanted to bark something back at me, but she didn't; she just held me.

I felt bad, but I was in no mood to chat or hang out with anyone, so I went to my room and stayed there all night. His mom made me cookies and tea to help comfort me. I don't think I slept an hour that night. I was so worried something was going to happen. Looking back now, it seems silly, but he hadn't been in a room alone overnight since his accident. Even when he was in the ICU and we weren't able to stay in the room with him, there was a twenty-four-hour nurse that did. He did great despite my worrying. When I got back to the hospital at 7:00 a.m., Jeff was still sleeping. He was very happy to see me that morning.

Journal update, Wednesday, August 17, 2011

Today was a great day! Jeff has been doing a lot better behaviorally the last few days. He seems less confused and seems to understand a little why he is in the hospital. He still doesn't want to be there, but he is beginning to understand why. He still doesn't think there is anything wrong with him, but he is starting to agree with us when we tell him some of the things he has trouble with. He has been much more mild tempered the last few days, which is a wonderful relief. He is a lot more compliant and is listening to more of what we tell him. He hasn't been at all aggressive in the last three days. I'm hoping that it will last!

Tonight is the third night in a row that he is sleeping on his own. He knows how to make phone calls from the room and calls me regularly if I'm not there. We are even able to leave him alone during the day. That takes a huge load off me because I was actually able to run some errands this morning. Of course, he's not completely alone; there are nurses and doctors around all the time, but we don't have to keep eyes on him 24/7 like we've had to for the last seven weeks. We put some signs up around the room to help him find things, and it seems to help a little. He has also learned how to call the nurses if he needs anything.

Today my cousins came to visit, and we played an entire game of Yahtzee. He needed a little help with figuring out what to roll, but he got the gist of the game and was able to do a lot of it on his own. Then this evening, we got a day pass and took him to his parents' house for dinner. Everything went great. We explained that he had to go back to the hospital afterward, and he was very concerned that we were going to be late. He kept asking what time it was. But we didn't have any problems getting him back

> or any problems at their house. He even helped clean the dishes when we were done eating. Since he did so well, we are going to attempt taking him home on a weekend pass. This will give him two more days in the hospital so he will get to be there until Tuesday. It also gives us a chance to see how he does and then ask the doctors and therapists questions if we have problems.

This seemed to be a turning point for Jeff. It was almost like something clicked in his head. He was much less angry all the time as well as much less aggressive toward me. When he did do something wrong, he was able to apologize for it. When Jeff didn't understand what his problems were, he didn't want to be in the hospital and didn't want to go to therapy. But now, it seemed that he was beginning to grasp that there was something wrong. He couldn't tell you what he needed to work on or what his problems were, but he understood that he did have difficulty with things that he thought he should be able to do. He was willing to accept help. I was told several times that once Jeff understood that there was something wrong, he would make quicker progress. That statement was very true. Once he recognized he had a problem, he was able to work on it.

I got to watch God work another miracle through a benefit that my friends and family put on for us during this time. They put together a benefit where people bought plates of food, and then there were live and silent auctions of items that had all been donated for us. It was incredible to watch how many people cared about us. Friends, family, and people in our community donated food and items for the auction. I was overwhelmed by the sheer number of people that came to the benefit and just bought plates of food. Every single item in the silent auction was sold. There were five or six long tables full of items that people bought to help us.

Then the live auction started. It was fun just to watch and listen to the auctioneer in action. My eyes began to get misty when I heard what the items were going for. Guided fishing tours, vacation packages, signed guitars, and other high-dollar items were all donated. People were bidding outrageous amounts on the items just to help us out. There were even a couple of items that were purchased and then donated back again to be sold so we made double the amount on a single item! On top of all of that, people were coming and handing me cash and checks just to help out. I was in awe.

God moved people to be so generous that it allowed me to stay home and take care of Jeff for as long as I needed to. I didn't have to worry about how I was going to pay the bills; it had all been taken care of. It was just one more thing that God showed me that I didn't have to worry about. "Can any of you by worrying add a single hour to your life?" (Matthew 6:27). "Cast your cares on the Lord and He will sustain you" (Psalm 55:22). I was continuing to learn that I had control over nothing, but I had no reason to worry because God has control over everything. Words really cannot express how grateful I am for all of the donations and generosity. I was completely overwhelmed with the love and kindness of others that night.

Preparing to Come Home

Journal update, Friday, August 19, 2011

Yesterday was not as good of a day as we have had all week. Jeff seemed to regress a little toward the evening. He was getting very confused again and agitated. He got upset and told everyone to leave. So we left. About an hour later, he decided to call me and tell me what a horrible person I am for dropping him off at the hospital and just leaving him there. He didn't want me to come back up, just wanted me to know that he was mad at me, and he hung up on me. The doctors warned us that he will go through phases, and it's normal for him to regress sometimes.

On the bright side, we are still planning on taking him home this weekend for a weekend pass. We will see how it goes. We are really worried that he won't want to go back to the hospital on Monday morning.

Jeff had one of the most difficult confabulations about this night. He was convinced that I had taken him to a different room. Even though the room looked exactly the same, he believed that it was a different room. Not only that, but he believed that I changed his room because I was angry with him and that I just left him there. He thought he was alone and that no one wanted to be around him. It didn't matter how hard I tried; I was unable to convince him otherwise.

After I left that night, Jeff called. "I just wanted to tell you what a horrible person you are."

"What are you talking about?" I asked, shocked.

"You left me!"

"Honey, I didn't just leave you, you told me to go. I was just doing what you asked."

"No, you left me here!"

"Jeff, I'll be back in the morning. You told me you wanted to be alone and that you wanted me to go, so I came home to get some sleep. I will be there with you first thing in the morning."

"NO! You left me!" Click.

I had done everything in my power to let him know that he wasn't alone in this and that I loved him no matter what. I didn't care what happened; I was his wife, and I was going to stick by his side. But it didn't matter. He wouldn't even let me come back to the hospital to explain things to him. He couldn't believe that I would leave him, and so he didn't want to see me.

I felt so alone that night. Tess and Brian were in my back yard mowing, and I wanted so badly to go out there and thank them, but all I could do was sit down on my bed and cry. I didn't know what to do to make him know how much I love him. I was alone in our house, just thinking about how alone he must feel sitting in that hospital room all by himself. I tried for months to convince him that I never changed his room that night and that I didn't just leave him there. It wasn't until five months after his accident that he finally believed me. He finally understood what a confabulation was and that he had them. We went through all the details of that night, and he finally believed that it was in his head.

The next day, Jeff finally got to come home for the weekend. There was a lot of preparation that went into this. I had to completely "Jeff-proof" the house, getting rid of all the rugs so he wouldn't trip. All knives, scissors, pills, and anything that Jeff could hurt me or himself with had to be locked up. It was like childproofing a house; only, he could reach the tall cabinets.

My mom and dad helped out a lot over this weekend. They took turns staying with us. To be honest, I was afraid to be home alone with Jeff. Not only was I worried that he might wander out the door while I wasn't looking, but I was afraid of him. He was still incredibly impulsive. If he wanted something and someone tried to stop him, he would push them out of the way. I was afraid that he would want to do something that he wasn't able to, and I would be what was getting in his way. I was afraid that he might try to hurt me in some way.

Thankfully, he never did. He would get angry and throw things, but he never hit me. The only times that he tried to was when he was at the first rehab hospital. He was much too slow then to really do any harm. Even though he was impulsive and didn't always know right from wrong, he was able to control himself in that.

As often happens with brain injury patients, he did not handle the change well. Even though he had been demanding to go home for weeks, once he got there, he was extremely agitated. It was one of those "be careful what you wish for" moments. I had wanted Jeff to be comfortable at the hospital so he wasn't miserable. However, that meant that he didn't want to be at home anymore.

Friday night and Saturday morning were really difficult. Saturday, my dad stayed with him while my mom took me out for a few hours. The time away seemed to be just what Jeff needed to adjust. By Saturday evening, he was doing much better. He just needed time to adjust to the change again. I suspect that he felt guilty for being unkind to me and felt that he drove me away. He was more pleasant after I returned.

I also learned over time that he was unhappy wherever he went. When he was in the hospital, he wanted to be at home. Once he went home, he wanted to be at the hospital. Later, he went to another rehab facility, and the cycle continued. He was just frustrated with his condition and blamed it on his location. I really had to try hard throughout this entire process not to take things personally. I continually had to remind myself that it was the brain injury causing things; it wasn't Jeff.

Despite the struggles, it was so wonderful to have Jeff home for a couple days. We got to do normal things again. Even though he still needed constant supervision, and my parents were staying with us to help, it was the closest thing to normal since his accident. He was still making progress, so I had hope that eventually he would be able to do normal things again without supervision. Little by little, Jeff was coming back.

MISCOMMUNICATIONS

Journal update, Thursday, August 25, 2011

Some people may be wondering why we are still trying to find a long-term facility for Jeff if he is doing okay at home. It's because he will be safer there, and he will be able to get more therapy than he would on an outpatient basis. The more therapy he is able to get, the quicker he is able to recover. It's better to have him in more intensive therapy for a shorter period of time than to spread it out over a longer period. The more therapy he can get now, the better because his brain is trying to fix itself more now than it will be later on in the process.

I also want to say thank you again for all the continued prayers and support. Today marks two months since Jeff's accident. It has been the longest two months of my life. However, I really appreciate everything everyone has done for us. It is encouraging when people tell me they are still praying because it lets me know that we haven't been forgotten. This is going to be a very long journey, and it helps to know that there are tons of people praying for and supporting us. So thank you.

Recovery from a brain injury is a very long and drawn-out process. As time passed, the recovery would slow down. The brain tries to heal itself the quickest at the beginning. Therefore, the more time that passed from the date of the injury, the less progress Jeff would make. It was imperative that he receive the most therapy as early on as possible while his brain was still trying to heal itself. That doesn't mean that if he hadn't received intensive therapy early on that he wouldn't have continued to recover. Although it does mean that he may not have recovered as much as he has. Jeff will likely continue to recover for the rest of his life. However, it will be much slower and less noticeable than what he was capable of early on.

I had another breakdown around this time. With emotions high, there was a lot of strain on my relationship with Jeff's family. Most of our disagreements were a result of misunderstanding each other's intentions. Our emotions were too charged to be able to think rationally all the time. We both wanted what was best for Jeff, but had different ideas for what that might be.

I had many family and friends offer their support early on. It was much needed, and I am very appreciative of it. Still, I knew that no matter how much support was offered while Jeff was in the hospital, once he came home, he was going to be my responsibility. I was going to be the one taking care of him. I knew that if he needed twenty-four-hour care for the rest of his life, eventually other people's ability to support would diminish over time.

I had many critical decisions to make in the first few weeks. And even later, there were decisions about what facility to take him to or what therapies he should receive. At times, these decisions were made that much more difficult because there were other people and opinions to consider. Thankfully, Jeff's family loves him dearly, but that meant they wanted to weigh in, and it caused tension, because I felt that I was the ultimate decision maker. Jeff and I were always blessed with wonderful in-laws. He got along great with my family, and I got along great with his. There was never any tension or problems with our families.

On this particular day, however, there was a miscommunication about a potential facility for Jeff. I completely blew it out of proportion, thinking they were keeping information from me for fear I might disagree with what they wanted to do. It was a complete misunderstanding, but I couldn't see that at the time. I was livid and felt like I just couldn't handle the drama with his family anymore. I couldn't handle Jeff's mood swings. I couldn't handle what life was going to be like when he came home. I was falling apart at the seams. I just didn't want to do it anymore. But that wasn't really an option; I had to find a way to put myself back together.

So, I finally decided to go to counseling. I have a master's degree in counseling, and I know how to help other people. I know what to say to others in bad situations and how to help them work through it. But it was a completely different story when that person was me. I couldn't work through it on my own. I couldn't see past what was right in front of me. I felt hopeless and deserted, even though I was surrounded by people that loved and cared about me.

I knew I had people that would listen and talk things through with me, but I just didn't feel comfortable pouring my heart out. I didn't want to share my hurt with my family because I knew that it hurt them to see me in pain, and I didn't want to make things worse for them. I didn't want to talk to my friends about it because they had their own struggles. I needed someone that was impartial, someone that didn't know me personally, and someone that could listen but also help me work through it. I didn't want advice. I needed someone that would help me find my own answers.

It didn't matter how strong I tried to be, at times I just needed to be able to break down. Counseling really helped me work through a lot of my issues and to talk openly about my fears. I was able to work through my frustrations with other people not understanding what it was like to be the wife of someone with a brain injury. I wasn't going anywhere. I made vows to Jeff on our wedding day, and I meant them. I don't care what other people thought I would or should do if Jeff didn't get better. I was not going to leave him. So, I had to figure out how to live with him again now that he was a different person. It was important for me to do this. I had been helping Jeff all this time, but I had to help myself as well. If I didn't, then I was going to be of no use to Jeff because I would burn myself out.

Like I said before, I was unable to see clearly what was happening because my mind was clouded by emotions that I wasn't able to process. I began to target all my unbridled emotions onto Jeff's family. As hard as they tried to be my ally and support, I didn't see it that way. I needed to aim my frustrations at someone, and they became the bull's eye.

I needed to sift through my emotions in counseling to help me see clearly again. I required guidance to discover healthier ways to cope with the numerous emotions that I had racing through my mind simultaneously. Once I had an outlet, I stopped trying to pin my anger on others and started accepting their help again. I became a better listener, and the miscommunications diminished.

Adjusting to Life at Home

Journal update, Friday, August 26, 2011

Today was Jeff's last day in the hospital for a while. He was a little agitated when he first got home but settled down much quicker than last weekend. He got to hang out with one of his friends at the house this evening while I went and had fun at Bunco right across the street. He did call and tell me he burnt the house down, and we would have to buy a new one. Thankfully, he was only joking, and there weren't any problems while I was gone.

Jeff really surprised me today. We were discussing the benefits of being in a facility full time versus being in outpatient therapy. Jeff actually said that he knows that therapy is good for him, that it will help him get better, and that he wants to get better! This is great on so many levels. He is realizing that there is something wrong with him, which means that he is able to work on those things intentionally. He is also willing to go to therapy and, thus, will get more out of it. I was actually shocked when he was talking. He just sounded so clearheaded. It didn't last all day, but he did have a very clear moment today, which is great!

Even though Jeff had made tremendous progress in a very short amount of time, the doctors were still skeptical about how much

Jeff would recover. They admitted that his recovery was proceeding much faster than expected but were still cautious that it could stop at any time. Throughout the journey, I received many encouraging stories in the guestbook from our online journal that gave me hope.

There was one from a coworker of Jeff's. She had been in a car crash, suffered a severe head trauma, and was in a coma for a week. She was told that she wasn't going to recover. But she did, and it has been fifteen years since her accident. She is gainfully employed and taking care of her two children. Another entry pointed me to Gabrielle Gifford, the senator that was shot in the head. She had just left rehab to vote on a bill in Washington, DC. Many other people would call to tell me of their encouraging stories.

It made me realize that this happens to more people than you would expect. In fact, two million people suffer from some kind of brain damage each year![8] Each one of those injuries manifests itself differently too. No wonder the doctors couldn't give me answers. They were only able to give me the statistics. They weren't able to factor in Jeff's personality or the fact that we serve a God of miracles.

I really learned through this entire process about how much we take things for granted. The smallest of accomplishments brought us the greatest joys. Something as simple as cleaning the house or going to the grocery store was a huge deal. All of those mundane tasks require a lot more energy and thought processes than I ever would have expected. It was wonderful when Jeff was able to accomplish a task, and I got to see the sense of accomplishment and pride on his face.

Walking through the grocery store for the first time was actually a lot of fun. We bought way too much stuff because Jeff was just picking things up and putting them in the grocery cart, but he was enjoying himself. He seemed amazed at how many items there were on the shelves. It was like watching a child in a candy store.

We also got to go to Sunday school together again. I had prepared everyone beforehand that Jeff would be coming. It was a little awkward because Jeff was self-conscious and didn't want to act like he had a brain injury (even though everyone already knew). I had also told the class that Jeff may or may not remember them. So our friends would come up to him and introduce themselves. Jeff pretended that he remembered people, and then he would ask me afterwards who they were.

Jeff was relearning where things were in the house, and I didn't have to follow him around everywhere anymore. He even made a pot of coffee on his own. The only thing I had to do was plug in the coffeemaker once he walked away. We recently bought a new coffeemaker that has a timer on it. So now, Jeff is able to get everything ready the night before, and it will start brewing his coffee when he gets up. Just the other day, I was getting my breakfast one morning and saw the light on indicating the timer had been set, and I smiled. He could do that all by himself; he didn't need my help anymore. It was just a small reminder of how far he has come.

Feeling Hopeless

Journal update, Thursday, September 1, 2011

I usually try to look on the bright side of this situation and talk about the positive things that are happening. But the reality of this situation is that living with Jeff is like living on an emotional roller coaster every day. One minute he is doing great, we are having great conversations, we are laughing together, and I look at him and feel hopeful. I think that everything is going to be okay; he is going to make a full recovery, and it's not going to take as long as the doctors think. But then out of nowhere, he is upset at me for something that he can't even tell me. I have no idea what I did, but he's mad at me, throwing things around the house and yelling, telling me that it's my fault that he's in this situation. I begin feeling hopeless and frustrated, like everything that I was just thinking gets thrown out the window because he's not doing any better. Then his outburst passes, and he's apologizing to me, telling me he didn't mean to take anything out on me. Then, the cycle starts all over again. All day long. There hasn't been a single day since he came home that this hasn't happened. I know it's part of the injury; he can't help it, and I'm not supposed to take it personally, but it's hard not to. So while you are praying for continued progress, please pray specifically for his mood swings.

All this time, I felt like I was trying to make things sound better than they were. I was exhausted mentally, physically, spiritually, and emotionally. Taking care of Jeff was taking everything out of me. I needed some encouragement and just felt like I wanted people to see a little bit of what I really was going through on a daily basis. This was no exaggeration; it was up and down all day long, every day. My body had been functioning at such high levels of adrenaline for so long that I think I was finally crashing. I was feeling depressed and hopeless and just didn't want to be on the roller coaster anymore. I wanted things to stabilize. I needed to start taking more time for myself so I could be rejuvenated and have the energy to keep going.

> Hey Casey—Thanks for your honesty. I can't imagine how hard that must be coming from your husband & how weary you must feel....the constant back & forth of his moods. I'm praying that during this time you can lean on the Lord for strength as you depend on Him for *everything...*
>
> —Kristen Parrish

> Hang in there. We are praying for you both. Your frustration is so understandable. Knowing that what Jeff is going through is to be expected does not make it any easier for you. You are one amazing person and your love for Jeff will get you through. God Bless and we will pray for help in a more specific way.
>
> —Sharon and Jim Koch

The therapists said that one of the reasons Jeff did so well at the hospital was due to the schedule and predictable routines. It was something I needed to implement at home, but was having a difficult time doing so. I hoped that it would help. I needed something to distract him from the constant emotional roller coasters he kept taking me on. If he was busy and could expect what was coming next, I hoped that would help with some of it. But by this point, I was getting worn out and didn't know what would really help him. I was at a point where I just expected this was going to be my life from now on.

The constant care Jeff needed was really wearing on me. I was also becoming anxious because I felt that he needed more therapy than just the few hours a week he was getting in outpatient therapy. He needed to live in a facility where he could get therapy through every day activities. I would get impatient, or afraid that he would do something incorrect, so I would just do things for Jeff.

I was desperately trying to find a live-in facility so Jeff could get the help he needed before it was too late and his brain wasn't remaking the connections they were at that time. I didn't want to just get rid of him so I didn't have to deal with the problems anymore. I knew that he needed help that I couldn't give him.

I took him to a tutoring facility that specialized in retraining the brain after brain injuries. They did an assessment on him that really put things into perspective for me. When you look at Jeff, he really doesn't seem like anything is wrong with him. When he's doing really well, and not in a bad mood, I start to get my hopes up too, thinking he's not that bad. However, this assessment proved otherwise.

The test scored things like memory, problem solving, math, reading, etc. In order to go back to work or be able to function in society independently, he would need to score around 50 percent. Out of the eight or so different sections, his highest percent was 11. Some were as low as 0.1 percent. While he'd made tons of improvement, he still had a long way to go.

That was a discouraging test and a reminder of just how far we still had to go in Jeff's recovery process. The people that ran the program told me that they couldn't guarantee that Jeff would get to the point where he could function independently in society. They did tell me that they would be able to improve his score and show measurable progress. I was so disheartened by that news. It brought to reality the fact that Jeff may never be able to return to work or a life that even resembled the life we lived before. I had accepted that fact, but I still hoped for more.

All the doctors, therapists, books, and statistics said that he would never be 100 percent back to where he was before the accident. However, they obviously didn't know my God and the miracles he can perform. I have seen him perform miracle after miracle in our lives over the last couple of months. I know that restoring Jeff to where he was before the accident is not too much to ask of my God. Jeff isn't a statistic; he is a child of the living God!

The only thing that I could do was trust in God. Again, I had no control over the situation, but God did. He already knew how our story was going to turn out. I just had to have faith that God would get us through it and give us the tools we needed to continue surviving.

Looking back now, I'm so glad that I didn't give up hope. I was right; they didn't know my God! My God could and did work miracles that were impossible by our standards. While it may not have been on my time frame, God worked impossible miracles, and Jeff was better not even a year after his accident, than the doctors thought he would be two years out.

After Jeff had been home a few weeks, I was able to get him into a live-in program. He would stay at the facility during the week and then come home on the weekends. It allowed him to get more intensive therapy than I could provide at home, but still have the benefit of being at home some of the time.

LETTING GO

Journal update, Monday, September 19, 2011

> Jeff went to the live-in facility this morning. He will be living there from Monday to Friday and then come home on the weekends. This isn't like the hospitals he has been at where I am there with him all day. I'm a little nervous about the whole thing because I'm not there to oversee that everything is being done correctly. Anyone that knows me knows I like to be in control, so this is scary for me. However, they have already called to assure me that he is doing fine. I'm really excited about it as well. We sat down and talked with the people in charge, and he is going to be getting a lot of help that I wasn't able to give him at home. He is going to learn a lot more independence than I would be able to give him. Independence in the sense that he will have to learn to do things for himself rather than me doing them for him.
>
> Please be in prayer that this will be good for him and that he will continue to make miraculous progress. Please pray for me that I will be okay with not being by his side 24/7 now.

God was teaching me a valuable lesson about control through this whole process. I have a type A personality and like to have control over everything around me. When I don't, my natural instinct is to pull things closer to me so I can feel like I do have more control over them. That was not possible during this time in my life. I had no control over Jeff's recovery. I did get to make a lot of decisions concerning it, and I was always by his side to oversee everything. Now that he was at this new facility though, I wasn't.

It was as though God was telling me that he would take care of everything. I was unwilling to give up control voluntarily, so he was taking more and more out of my control. I didn't have a choice in the matter. God wanted to teach me that he could handle it all. It doesn't matter how much I plan or try to control the situations around me, ultimately, it was in his hands, not mine. I am a very stubborn person, and I just didn't want to let go. So God had to take me to a place where I didn't have a choice. Once I stopped fighting though and just let him take care of things, I had a sense of freedom. It felt like a huge weight was lifted off me. I had been carrying around the stress of the entire situation. I was carrying Jeff's stress for him because he had no worries. I was carrying the stress of how his recovery would go. I was carrying the stress of what to do in every situation. Once I let it go, I was so relieved. Regardless of what I thought, I didn't have control over any of those situations.

I know that I prayed and asked for others to pray that God would take care of things throughout the entire journey, but I was still fighting for control. Even after this realization, I still fought some, but I would quickly be reminded that it wasn't my battle to fight. It did make things a lot easier for me when I wasn't trying to control everything and just trusted God to take care of it.

Now, it is a lot easier to recognize when I am trying to take control again. I have come to a place where I am all right not knowing what will happen. I am able to trust that God will provide; he will take care of us. I have a lot more peace in my life now. I can now recognize when God gives me the next piece of the puzzle, and I try to finish it. I can now stop myself; I can take the next piece and say, "thank you," instead of, "where's the one after that?" It doesn't mean I don't still try to make plans for my life, but I'm a lot more open to the changes that may happen to those plans. I'm content with the fact that the plans I have may not happen at all.

I want to note that just because God granted me peace, it doesn't mean that I didn't still feel sorrow. I was hurting deeply in more ways than I thought were possible. I cried, I hurt, I called out to God; even now, tears still come to my eyes when I think about everything we went through. However, in the midst of it all, I had peace. I knew that God would get me through it, and he calmed me. He granted me the wisdom to know that he would get me through everything. I knew that I wasn't alone.

During this stage, I also learned that Jeff wasn't happy anywhere. When he was in the rehab hospitals, he wanted to go home. When he finally came home, he wanted to go back to the hospital. He would tell me that he didn't like living with me because he was such a burden. Then, when he was at rehab during the week and at home on the weekends, he wanted to be home all the time. This was very difficult on me because I wanted him to be happy. I wanted him to like where he was. When he complained about living away from home, I had to remind myself that he didn't want to be at home when he was there either. It was a constant struggle to know what was best for him and to remember that he wanted to make decisions based on his feelings at the moment, not based on what would help him get better.

After just three months, as Jeff continued to make progress and get better, it became a lot harder for me to see the progress on a daily basis. He did continue to progress, but it was harder to recognize. Instead of learning to walk and talk, he was learning to comprehend sentences or follow directions. I had to look closer to see what he had accomplished. Sometimes, I had to take a step back and look at where he had been a week ago to notice how well he was doing that day. This was good; it just took effort on my part not to feel like he was getting stuck where he was in his progress. I had to continually check that he was still progressing.

I was also trying to transition back into the role of a wife instead of a mother. That was extremely hard to do. There were times when Jeff did still need to be mothered and needed lots of instruction. There were other times, though, when I needed to let go and allow Jeff to make his own choices. He no longer needed the constant supervision he once did. I had to adjust to my ever-changing role. I had to remind him to utilize the tools he was learning to use to help him with his everyday tasks. I had to let go of my mindset that he was this person with a brain injury that I would have to take care of forever. I had to embrace the new man my husband was becoming and start treating him like my husband again.

Adjusting to the New Normal

Journal update, Monday, October 17, 2011

I may not understand why God has allowed something like this to happen to us, but it has been amazing to watch him work through it. For some reason, this past week has been very emotional for me. I've been thinking a lot about the first few days after Jeff's accident. I didn't know if he was going to live, and if he did, what kind of life he would have. I thought I had given up all my hopes and dreams for what I expected my life to be. My life was turned completely upside down. But now, life is beginning to resemble something a little more normal. Instead of wondering if Jeff is going to wake up and what kind of care he is going to need, we are looking at what his abilities are. Now the questions seem to be more of "when" instead of "if." We are beginning to discuss Jeff's job abilities and when he will be able to return to work. Of course, it's still a long way off, but it's possible now. Just a few months ago, I didn't know if it would be. I have a whole new appreciation for life and the little things. It's been wonderful to watch God work in so many ways throughout this process. Anyone who works with Jeff that is familiar with brain injuries still is amazed at his progress. Thank you for all your continued prayers. I know that God is working miracles because we ask and we believe, and I know that he will continue.

I kept hoping and waiting for things to return to normal. I realized, however, that if I kept waiting for the Jeff I knew to come back, I wouldn't be able to enjoy the new Jeff that I received. I learned that I couldn't hold on to the past but had to discover how to live with Jeff as he is now. It was a key adjustment that I had to make in order to make our marriage work. Had I held onto who Jeff used to be, I would have always been disappointed. An important part of a marriage is making adjustments and compromises; this was just another one of those compromises on a larger scale.

Even as Jeff was recovering and hope was returning, I still had a lot of ups and downs personally. There would be times that I was fine, looking forward and rejoicing with Jeff's progress. There were other times, though, where I would have flashbacks. Even now, I still struggle with that. They come out of nowhere. I will start picturing the night of the accident and how Jeff looked being carried in on the ATV. Other times, it's the first few days at the hospital and the emotional roller coaster I was on. It wasn't just the images in my head; all the emotions that I felt at the time come flooding back. It will happen at church in the middle of a sermon, when I'm driving in the car, and even when I'm talking with someone about something completely unrelated. The pictures and emotions just flood my mind, and I have to hold back the tears because the people around me don't understand what's going on. Sometimes this would last for days at a time, and I would just be a mess. Other times, it would last for a couple minutes and then not happen for a couple weeks.

It is still really difficult to talk about. I can talk about Jeff's current progress usually without any problems, but if someone asks me about early on, it can be very difficult to discuss. Writing this book has been a huge struggle. In a way, it has been therapeutic because I got to think through everything in a safe environment. In another way, it has been difficult to relive the experience. Many parts of this book were written a paragraph at a time. I would start writing and just get too upset to continue, so I would have to walk away.

I was discussing my flashbacks with Jeff and the difficulties it caused me. He made a comment about not understanding why it was so difficult because he wasn't having a hard time with it. Jeff has no memory for the first two months after the accident. He remembers the night of the accident up until about an hour or so before it happened. Then he has no memory until the third hospital he was in. Even then, it is only vague memories of people or a few events that happened. I had to remind him that it wasn't difficult for him because he didn't have to deal with the ups and downs that I went through while he was unconscious. Then after he awoke, he has no memory of the difficulties he had in relearning everything needed to function in daily life. His struggles dealt more with the difficulties he had on a daily basis and not with memories of the past. I, on the other hand, had to learn to cope with both.

I was reading a book about a missionary in Asia and the trials he had. While his trials were much different from mine, the truths apply to my situation.

> In some way, which I still do not really understand, the trying of our faith works patience and hope into the fabric of our Christian lives. No one, I am convinced, will follow Jesus very long without tribulation. It is His way of demonstrating His presence. Sufferings and trials—like persecution—are a normal part of the Christian walk.[9]

This suffering wasn't happening to us because we were bad people, or because we were being punished for something. We weren't immune to it because we are Christian. Jesus promised that "in this world you will have trouble" (John 16:33). I couldn't blame God. I needed to lean on him to get me through the difficult times that he promised would come into our lives. I could not think I was different than any other Christian who has endured hardship.

Jeff's doctor had taken him off his medications that controlled his mood because he wanted to change them, but he didn't just want to switch. He wanted to see what they were doing for him before he changed them. Therefore, he decided to take him off all medications and see what happened. I was so worried about this because he already had a lot of mood swings, and I didn't want them to be worse. However, God was still in control. Taking him off the medications really seemed to help Jeff. His moods stabilized, and he seemed to be able to control himself a little better. It was like God said, "Let me handle this."

This was also a time that helped me to see Jeff from an outsider's perspective. I wasn't living with Jeff day in and day out anymore, so I would only see him for a couple hours during the week and on the weekend. This is the amount of time that most of his family had been spending with him leading up to this point. From this outside perspective, Jeff seemed to be doing a lot better than he actually was. I didn't see his day-to-day difficulties and frustrations. When he would come home on the weekends, he seemed to be on his best behavior because he was trying to prove to me that he was all right to come home.

However, once he did come home full-time, I realized that he had not made quite the amount of progress that I thought he had. While he did make tremendous progress, it was a dramatic difference living with him full-time and living with him part-time. It helped me understand more why other people didn't understand why I was so protective of him. Being around him all the time allowed me to see what he was really like, not what he was like when he was trying to impress someone.

After 4 months, Jeff was finally ready to be at home full-time and stay there. Outpatient therapy was still needed, but the constant therapy from the live-in program no longer was. Not only that, but Jeff was making such wonderful progress that we could confidently say that he was capable of returning to work in some capacity. I was able to enroll him in a vocational rehab program to help him go back to work.

This was huge because we finally had a goal. It wasn't just a matter of "wait and see" how well he will get. We were working toward him going back to work. It was still a long ways off, but it was in the future. Jeff was really excited to be back home and was motivated to keep working hard and doing his therapy so he could continue to get better.

Even as Jeff was showing marked improvements and was becoming more himself, it was still hard living with him. He was a different person. In some ways, the changes were good. He was much more affectionate than he was before. He really appreciated me after the accident and was very grateful for me and everything that I had done for him. He was more vocal about his feelings and gratitude for me.

In other ways though, the changes were harder to cope with. While he wasn't angry all the time, throwing things, and yelling at me anymore, he was much more dependent. I have had a hard time adjusting to our new roles as husband and wife. I have had to be much more protective of him than I used to be. He was just childlike. It wasn't necessarily a bad thing, but it was different. He was also a lot more sensitive than he used to be. I had to learn how to speak to him again. When I got upset and normally would lose my temper, I had to learn to control myself and not yell or say something I would regret later. When I used to say something that he would just shrug off, after the accident, he couldn't move past it. If I said something out of anger, it would fester in him, and he couldn't let go of it.

After her husband's brain injury, Barbara Cooper realized that:

> You will not be able to move on with your journey in your life, staying stuck in your turmoil, if you refuse to let go of the old to make room for the new. Acceptance of the

> situation is the key that will unlock your heart to bring about a new beginning. Acceptance of the situation does not mean that you have given up hope of the situation becoming better.[10]

I needed to stop waiting for things to go back to the way they were. I needed to learn who Jeff is now and begin a life with the new him. While he may make a full recovery, he will never be 100 percent who he was before, and I needed to start my life with him as he is now. I had to stop waiting for Jeff to come back and enjoy the Jeff I had now.

Typically, six months after the accident, doctors say that people with a brain injury will have made 80 percent of their progress. After that, it takes another eighteen months for the remaining 20 percent of what they will recover to come back. Once we hit the six month mark, Jeff was doing remarkably well. That's when I noticed other problems start to emerge. He began to struggle with depression. It wasn't a terrible depression, but I noticed remarkable differences in his mood. He wasn't as moody as he had once been, but he was just down the majority of the time.

Jeff really enjoyed his job, and sitting around the house, unable to work, was not his idea of a good time. It became very difficult to motivate him to do anything. Everything I suggested sounded boring to him. He knew that whatever he did, he would get bored with it soon, so he would rather just sit on the couch and watch TV. It was difficult for me because I didn't like to see him like that. I felt guilty much of the time because I was substitute teaching and gone for most of the day. So Jeff would be home alone by himself for the majority of the day with no way to leave the house to go do anything. I felt like it was my fault he was depressed, but I was assured that it is a very common reaction after a brain injury. Even when I was home, he still didn't want to do anything. I had to remind myself not to take things personally and just do what I could to help Jeff.

To make matters worse, he didn't know how to have fun anymore. He used to be a very social guy and loved to be around people. He was always the life of the party. After his accident though, he was not confident in social situations. He wasn't able to do some of the things that he did before, and he was insecure. He no longer wanted to hang out with friends or go to social gatherings that we once enjoyed doing every chance we got. When we did go somewhere, he usually wanted to leave very early. It took a lot of coaxing and encouragement from friends, but he finally started coming out of his shell again. He is definitely not as outgoing as he used to be, but he is more comfortable in social settings now.

A brain injury is just like other injuries in that there will always be lingering problems as a result of the injury. If a professional baseball player were to injure his shoulder, he may recover and seem fine. He may even be able to play baseball again, but if the injury is significant enough, he may never be able to play professionally again. The baseball player could go through life and never have any problems with his shoulder until he tries playing baseball or doing something that uses his shoulder in a significant way.

The same is true for a brain injury. Even after Jeff had recovered significantly, to the point that others didn't notice a difference, he still had lingering problems. Years down the road, he may be able to get through life just fine without having problems. However, if he were to try something new or more challenging than he is used to, he could have difficulty doing so or may not be able to do it at all. Just because Jeff no longer shows symptoms of his brain injury, doesn't mean that he is healed 100 percent back to how he was prior.

Provisions and Miracles

Journal update, Thursday, August 11, 2011

I just want to brag on how awesome my God is for a little bit. He has been providing for us for almost the last seven weeks in ways I can't even believe. Well, first of all, Jeff is still with us! Beginning with Jeff's initial injury, all he had were a few cuts and bruises other than the head injury. There were no broken bones, and all his scrapes healed before he even woke up. He has made progress almost every single day. The doctors and therapists are amazed. He is providing financially in ways I never could have even hoped for. We have had, so far, four and a half weeks of completely free rehab for Jeff. He is providing for our basic financial needs for living. I had to quit my job to be able to be there for Jeff, so God is providing everything right now. He is sustaining me emotionally, physically, spiritually, and is basically just carrying me through this. He has provided support for us through all of this. I know Jeff still has a very long way to go, but I also know that my God is bigger than anything that could ever be thrown at us, and he will get us through it. I don't know what the future is going to hold, but I know that whatever it holds, it will bring God glory, and he is somehow going to make something amazing out of all of this. I want to thank each and every one of you for allowing God to use you to minister to us in all

> the many ways that you have. You have no idea how much it means and helps.

"Even in your old age and gray hairs I am he, I am he who will sustain you. I have made you and I will carry you; I will sustain you and I will rescue you" (Isaiah 46:4). The most important lesson (and there have been many) that I have learned through this process is that God is sovereign. He knows that we will endure difficulties, but he promises that he will help us through them. It has been absolutely incredible to watch how God worked through everything that happened. Not only did he work miracle after miracle, but he did exactly what he promised in this verse, he *carried* me, he *sustained* me, he *rescued* me. God gave me strength and encouraged me when I thought I couldn't take it anymore. During a time when it would have been easy to shut down, go into a deep depression, and give up, God rescued me and gave me a peace that surpasses all understanding (Philippians 4:7). I truly believe that I never would have made it through this without God's help.

I wanted to take some time to share some of the wonderful things that God has done throughout this journey. God's provision in all of these things was amazing to watch. There is no way that Jeff would be doing as well as he is without God. To go through this journey and not give God credit would just be absurd. Jeff has made so much progress in such a short period that it is impossible by human standards. It is possible only by God and the miracles that he performed through this journey.

In his book *Second Guessing God: Hanging on When you Can't See His Plan*, Brian Jones describes two kinds of miracles. The first type are instantaneous miracles. These are the obvious ones where God heals someone or does something instantly that is unexplainable. The second type are perseverance miracles. In this type of miracle, God gives his supernatural strength to persevere through a problem that we could never trudge through on our own.[11] God performed both types in both me and Jeff. God granted me his supernatural strength and perseverance to make it through this trial. I will share below some of the instantaneous miracles he performed.

Let me share just a few of the highlights of the wonderful ways God provided for us. Jeff had no insurance. He was working, but he had only been at his job a couple months and didn't qualify for their insurance yet. He obviously wasn't going to be going back to work any time soon. I eventually had to quit my job to take care of him. We had an income of $0. We did rack up quite a large medical bill at the hospital in the ICU for twelve days. However, once he left, God provided in so many ways just financially. I will get to the other amazing provisions shortly.

When Jeff was discharged from ICU, he was transferred to an acute rehab hospital. He was able to stay there and get medical attention, medications, food, and therapy at absolutely no cost to us for three whole weeks. Normally, this facility doesn't even take patients on a charity basis, but because we knew one of the head guys that worked there, they were able to make an exception. He stopped working there shortly after Jeff left. Had Jeff not recovered at the pace he did, that spot would not have been available.

From there, he was transferred to a second rehab facility, also in San Antonio, for four weeks. Again, because of someone we knew, at absolutely no cost to us. While there, not only did he get treatment, but they also held a group therapy session for families of people with brain injuries, also at no cost. I finally was getting some help for myself and met some other wives who finally understood what I was going through. When I got to the point that I realized I needed individual counseling to cope with my own struggles, that was also provided for me.

It wasn't until nine weeks after Jeff's accident that he was finally discharged to go home. Had he been discharged just a week sooner, he would not have been safe enough to be at home. Of course, he still needed therapy, so God provided outpatient therapy for him three days a week. Not only was it free, but it was only five minutes away from our house. So, I no longer had to drive an hour to see Jeff every day. In the meantime, my parents put on a fundraiser for us to help pay just the normal bills of everyday life. It was the biggest fundraiser that the venue had ever done and raised more money than they had ever raised before at one event. God allowed me to be able to stay home with Jeff, not to have to worry about being able to work and still be able to pay our bills. All of these things in themselves were amazing, but the fact that all of them happened is nothing short of God's amazing provision for his children.

Now for the provisions and miracles that didn't have to do with money... Jeff was thrown from a four-wheeler and hit his head on a tree. Just the fact that he lived is a miracle in itself. He was knocked unconscious immediately. He had some cuts and bruises, but other than the brain injury, he had sustained no other major injuries, no broken bones, nothing. Not even his skull was fractured. He had bleeding in the brain, which normally causes massive swelling. Swelling in the brain can be very dangerous because there is nowhere for it to expand. Jeff's swelling was so minimal that they didn't even consider it swelling. He never needed surgery.

God provided a huge network of friends and family for support. Our neighbors and people from our small group at church helped out at home. People walked our dogs, cleaned our house, and made meals for me. People took turns staying the night with Jeff at the hospital and even with me at home the first few nights. I had people that I was able to talk to or just cry with. There were people that prayed over us when I wasn't able to.

God's timing through this entire process was perfect. The accident happened over the summer, so I had two months to figure out what I was going to do before I had to return to work. Since I had opted for annual payroll, I still got a paycheck through August even though I wasn't working. Both Jeff's sisters and his brother-in-law were also teachers, so they were able to help more than if they had been working. By the time school started, I didn't need as much help with him. We were both young and healthy prior to the accident, so we were better able to cope with it—Jeff, because his mind was able to heal faster than if he had been older, and me, because I still had the energy of a twenty-six-year-old. We didn't have any children to worry about yet. There was only a short window of time that Jeff would have been able to go to the first rehab facility, and it was worked out perfectly for him to go. The outpatient facility that Jeff attended when he finally came home was a brand-new facility. They were just getting started and had not gotten approval to charge their patients yet. So his therapy there was free. Had it taken any longer, we would have had to pay for his outpatient therapy, which would have cost $200/day.

The speed of Jeff's recovery was a miracle in itself. We were told time and again that he was making amazingly speedy progress. When I prayed specifically for God to start working miracles, he made such significant progress overnight that it caught the attention of his therapists. The amount of recovery Jeff made was also a miracle. The doctors didn't know if he was going to be able to function independently let alone go back to work. I was told time and again that his recovery would be at least a two-year process. Even after that time, he probably wouldn't be where he was before the accident. His recovery was so quick that by six months, he was past where the doctors expected him to be at two years. He still has more recovery to go, but I know that God will continue working miracles.

One of the trademarks of brain injury is impulsiveness. Typically, people with a brain injury are less likely to think through decisions and are more likely to put themselves in dangerous situations because of it. Jeff has had the opposite happen. Because of his injury, he is more careful than he used to be. He is cautious and doesn't want to put himself in any situation that would put him at risk for another brain injury. Jeff used to be impulsive before his accident, so this was a huge worry of mine.

I could only imagine what it was going to look like for him to be even more impulsive than he was before. God took care of that for us though. We prayed for it not to be an issue, I prayed specifically that it would be better than it was before, and God healed that part of the brain, precisely the way that I prayed he would.

For a long time, it was not certain whether Jeff was going to be able to work in any capacity, let alone be able to go back to doing what he did before his accident. Even if we thought that he could go back, what company would take the risk of letting him try it out, not knowing if he could even perform the duties of the job? However, our God is the God of miracles! Eight months after Jeff's accident, he returned to the job that he was doing before at the same company! Not only that, but they allowed him to try it out and go back slowly to make sure he was able to perform the functions of his job and that he was able to sustain the mental energy he needs to be there all day. He started out at just ten hours a week, and over the course of several months, was finally able to go back to work full-time!

People could call this coincidence; they could say he is just making faster recovery than normal, but I know the truth. It is possible for a few of these things to occur and call it coincidence. But there is no way that all of them could have happened on their own. God's hand was in everything. He watched over and protected us through the entire process and will continue to do so for the rest of our lives. He made sure that Jeff had the right doctors and hospitals, and God healed my husband beyond what is capable in human standards.

Happy Endings

> Journal update, Thursday, November 24, 2011
>
> Happy Thanksgiving, everyone! I sure do have a lot to be thankful for this year. First, I'm thankful for my miracle of a husband and how well he is doing. Tomorrow will be five months since his accident. He still continues to make progress. Everything we have been through has really put life into perspective for both of us and has caused us to be much more appreciative of what we have and of each other. I am thankful for all our family and friends, all the love and support you have shown us, and for the opportunities to see how many people truly care about and love us. We are blessed. I am thankful for miracles, many that I have been able to witness over these last five months. I am thankful for a loving, merciful, and wonderful God who has not let us down and continues to provide for and care for us. I am thankful that I get to spend Thanksgiving with Jeff and our family. I am thankful for all the prayers that you have prayed for us and that they have been answered. I am thankful for the time that I get to spend with Jeff. I am thankful for a new outlook on life and that it has been put into perspective for me. I am thankful for the things in life that really matter and that I am able to let go of the things that don't. This Thanksgiving, look around you, and be thankful for what God has blessed you with

I realize that not all stories end this way. Not everyone has a miraculous recovery the way my husband has. Jeff and I had a friend in our small group who was battling with cancer. She was Jeff's age and had two young children. She passed away. If ever there was a woman who lived her life for God, it was her. I felt so guilty. While I was grateful that God granted a miracle for Jeff, I didn't understand why he wouldn't do the same for her. I almost didn't go to her funeral because I felt like I was rubbing it in that Jeff got better and she didn't. It was a huge internal struggle for me. I still don't understand why God chose to heal Jeff and not our friend. I may never understand, but God does. Nothing happens by accident, and God can see the entire picture; we can only see the part that we are in.

Everyone's recovery is different. Everyone's story is different. While I believe in miracles and I know that God performed many in my husband and in our lives, I also recognize that God doesn't answer everyone's prayers in the same way. Miracles were part of God's plan for our lives; they are not part of his plan for everyone's lives. I encourage you to pray for miracles if that is what you want, but if God doesn't grant them, then ask for the strength to get through it. Just because he doesn't perform miracles, doesn't mean he won't comfort you through your struggles.

Despite the fact that a terrible thing happened, I am grateful for the good that has come from our suffering. I like how Barbara Johnson views suffering:

> I like to compare suffering to making a cake. No one sits down, gets out a box of baking powder, eats a big spoonful, and says, "Hmmm, that's good!" And you don't do that with a spoonful of shortening or raw eggs or flour, either. The tribulation and suffering in our lives can be compared with swallowing a spoonful of baking powder or shortening. By themselves, these things are distasteful and they turn your stomach. But God takes all of these ingredients, stirs them up, and puts them in His own special oven, thinking *Surely the cake must be done by now.* But not yet,

> no, not yet. What really matters is that the cake is *baking* and the marvelous aroma is filling the house.[12]

I know that God is sovereign and in control of everything that happens in our lives. He will never let me endure something that he knows I couldn't handle with his help. Even the pain endured by Job was approved by God. Satan had to ask permission from God, and "The Lord said to Satan, 'Very well, then, everything he has is in your power, but on the man himself do not lay a finger'" (Job 1:12). Satan's intentions were to turn Job away from God by inflicting numerous tragedies upon him, but God knew Job's heart and knew that Job would never turn from God. Job's tribulations brought him closer in his relationship with God and brought God glory.

In his book *Handle with Prayer*, Charles Stanley writes:

> Most of the time we pray, "Get me out of here!" We want to avoid suffering and difficulty. When we *do* run into a trial or difficulty, we ask God to change our circumstances so we can serve Him better and love Him more... We're more intent on getting out of our circumstances than we are on finding out what great things God wants to show us. But the Father never allows difficulty just for the sake of difficulty—there is always a higher purpose involved.[13]

When Jeff's accident first happened, all I cared about was being done with the suffering. I didn't want to go through what God was taking me through, and I cried out to God to "fix" everything. But, if he had answered that prayer, I would have missed out on all the blessings that I received from the trials.

God was fully aware of the pain that he allowed me to endure. It does not mean that God wanted to cause me pain or that he caused it himself. There are many reasons why God may have allowed this tragedy in our lives. He could have been teaching us a lesson. It could be a punishment for something we did. God could have been protecting us from something even worse happening in the future. Or it could simply be a result of living in a fallen world, a world that is not what God intended.

I could have questioned God and asked why he would allow this to happen to us. I could have laid out for him all the good things I have done or pointed out what a devoted Christian I am. I could have listed off all the good Christian things I did. But in the end, it doesn't matter. Bad things happen to everyone. Just because I am a Christian, does not make me immune to tragedies in this life. Jesus himself suffered. We have to remember that "Only *after* the cross comes the resurrection. Only *after* the cross comes glory."[14] There would be no resurrection if Jesus had not endured the pain of crucifixion. I just had to trust that God is in control, no matter what he allows to happen; I had to trust him, turn to him, and lean on him.

The Bible tells about the story of Joseph, who had eleven brothers. Those brothers planned to kill him but decided to sell him into slavery instead. They were so sure they would never see him again; they told their father he was killed by a wild animal. Yet years after Joseph's brothers sold him into slavery, they were reunited. At that time, he was a ruler under Pharaoh and was basically given control over everything in Pharaoh's kingdom. He was number two in all of Egypt. He told his brothers, "You intended to harm me, but God intended it for good to accomplish what is now being done" (Genesis 50:20). During that time, between being sold to slavery and being reunited with his family, Joseph endured many trials. He would do good and be rewarded with punishment. Throughout it all though, he remained faithful to God. Just like Joseph, I had to trust that somehow God would use this for good, and it would bring him glory.

"And we know that in all things God works for the good of those who love Him, who have been called according to His purpose" (Romans 8:28). Note that God does not say everything *will* be good. He says that everything is worked out *for* our good. That is a huge difference. So many people mistakenly believe that if God really loved us, he wouldn't let bad things happen to us. This thinking is simply not true. However, God does take the bad things and turn them into good. "God's providence means he is always working behind the scenes, outside of our view, to provide us with *something*, even when we don't understand what's happening at the time."[15]

There have been so many good things that have come from this suffering in our lives. Let me share just a few. I got to see how many people truly care for and love us. I got to watch God work miracle after miracle. I now live with a walking miracle. I was able to fully trust in and rely on God to get me through the hardest time of my life.

Now that Jeff is getting better, our relationship is better than it has ever been. It has caused us to grow closer together and have a much deeper appreciation for each other. Jeff is more appreciative of the life that he has regained and is so grateful to me for everything that I did for him.

It has brought other people closer to God. I have a friend who is an atheist who told me that there has to be something to prayer because there is no way that Jeff should be doing as well as he is. Life has been put in perspective, and we don't have to worry about the little things anymore because we know that God will take care of them.

God has brought me closer to him. In the midst of the darkest, most uncertain times in my life, I had peace. I have joy and peace. I am more patient and kind than I was before. I am more understanding and compassionate. I am more worry-free than I have ever been in my life during a time when there is no clear path for my future. A weight has been lifted from my shoulders, and I can focus on letting Christ shine through me instead of obsessing over the rules and checklists of being a Christian. I am free!

Once Jeff was working part-time, and I knew it was safe for me to go back to work again, I had complete trust in God. It was nearing summertime, and I was looking for a teaching position to start work in the fall. I kept praying that God would bring something along, but prayed that if teaching wasn't what God wanted for me, to guide me in the right direction.

I applied for several teaching positions, but didn't get a call back from any of them. The Wednesday of the last week of school, I prayed on my way to work, "God, I want to be able to enjoy the summer and not have to worry about finding a job. If it's in your plan for me to be a teacher, please provide a job before the school year ends so I don't have to worry about it all summer. If not, I trust you, and if teaching isn't where you want me to be, then please show me where you want me."

That afternoon, I had a voice mail from a private Christian school. They wanted me to come in for an interview. The previous week, I had driven by the school and dropped off my resumé. I hadn't even applied for the job yet, but they wanted to see me. The interview was scheduled for the following week.

I went in, assuming I was being interviewed for a teaching position, but when I got there, they had another position in mind. They wanted me to be the assistant director of their before-and-after-school program as well as the summer program. It was something I never would have considered and never would have applied for. They told me to take my time and pray about it.

I took a couple weeks to pray about it, and discuss it over with Jeff. Because it was a private school, the money wasn't going to be anywhere near what I would get as a teacher in a public school, and I had to work summers. As I continued to pray about it and share my hesitations with God, one by one, he confirmed this was where I was supposed to be. Jeff was doing great at his job and was expecting to be working full-time himself soon. We decided that, with his income increasing to full-time, that we would be able to make up the difference with my lower than expected income. So I accepted the job.

Then, we found out that Jeff wasn't going to be able to get full-time work like we expected. Before the accident, when Jeff was unemployed, I was a nervous wreck. I was constantly breathing down Jeff's neck to get a job, and we fought all the time about it. This time, I wasn't a nervous wreck. Instead, I became excited… it was a chance for God to show once again how he knows my every need better than I do.

I started praying that if God didn't want us to make any more money, then he would show us how to cut back even further than we already had so we could make ends meet. It took another four months, but not only did Jeff end up getting to work full-time, he was given a raise! Throughout those four months, instead of panicking, I had peace, and I trusted God to provide. God once again showed that he knew what I needed better than I did. "The Lord Himself goes before you and will be with you; he will never leave you nor forsake you. Do not be afraid; do not be discouraged" (Deuteronomy 31:8). Because I placed my trust in him, he blessed me with a job that I never would have found on my own, that I absolutely love, and Jeff is able to work full-time, making more money than we expected.

Conclusion

On June 20, five days before Jeff's accident, I wrote in my personal journal. I was having trouble sleeping that night because I was going back and forth with a lot of decisions that I needed to make. I decided to get up and pray about it through journaling. I had just finished my first year of teaching and really enjoyed what I did. However, I did not enjoy where I worked. I had been trying to find another teaching job somewhere else but was having no luck. With the budget cuts that were happening, schools just weren't hiring new teachers. Before teaching, I worked in sales, and my old boss had been trying to hire me back since the day I quit. So, I was battling with the decision to return to the same school and be miserable for another nine months or return to my previous job in sales. I wrote about it, asking God for guidance.

I went back and forth, telling God all the ideas that I had of how he could make things work out for us. Then I wrote, "I start reading this book I've been reading and get to this sentence. James 4:3, 'You ask and do not receive, because you ask with wrong motives, so that you may spend it on your pleasures.' Um, dagger to the heart!" I realized that I had been telling God what I wanted instead of asking what his will was. I was asking for his help but only to further my own pleasures. I finally broke down and prayed, "I want your will, but you have to show me how to get there. God, I need steps. Even if it's just the next one, I need to know what to do next. What do I do next?"

Then, five days later, none of my plans mattered anymore. God's answer was, "Focus on today. Follow me. Trust me. I will take care of you." Please don't mistake what I am saying. I am not saying that God caused Jeff's accident. I am not saying that Jeff's accident happened because I prayed about something. However, when God's children are ready to be broken for him, to serve him, to seek and do his will, their lives will never be the same.

I was finally at a place where I was ready to listen and receive what God had in store for me. God's timing is perfect. I believe that Jeff would have been in some sort of accident regardless, but God allowed it to happen when I was most receptive to him. He allowed it to happen when I was in a place spiritually that I could handle something that traumatic and life changing. I know that this experience would have changed me regardless of where I was spiritually or mentally. It's not possible to experience something that life changing and not come out different. But I also understand that I changed for the better because I was receptive to what God wanted me to see and learn through it.

I was a follower of Christ before, but I finally came to a place where I was willing to die to myself to follow him. When that happens, your life has to change. You cannot truly follow Christ without changing the way you live. I have made many life changes since becoming a Christian, but I was still holding something back. I was still holding back control. I wanted to have the ultimate say in where I went and what decisions I made. I wanted to make a plan for my life and follow it. "It's much easier to speak about following Jesus when you are making a general statement without any specific commitments. But the most obvious and basic definition of following Jesus will mean making some significant life changes."[16]

This does not mean that God wants to make your life hard or wants you to endure difficult times. He takes no pleasure in your pain. However, we are a stubborn people, and sometimes we need big events to get our attention. He wants to be first in our lives, and to be first, we have to give up what we are putting before God. "He made no compromises when he came and gave his life up for you, and he takes no compromises now as he asks you to do the same."[17] I was finally ready to follow Jesus wherever he wanted me to go no matter what the cost.

If you really want to follow Christ, you have to understand that. There will be trials; there will be difficulties. When you are ready to truly follow Christ, pray and ask God to change you to make you more like him no matter what that looks like. Then, be ready for some serious changes. It will be hard. It will hurt. But on the other side, there is joy beyond what anyone could ever describe to you and peace greater than you could ever have imagined.

For a while, I said that while I was grateful for the good that has come from this, I would never want to go through it again. However, knowing what I know now and seeing how much better it is on the other side, I can embrace whatever tragedies and struggles that lie ahead. I'm not saying that I would want to go through it again, but I know now that I am able to get through it. I have seen God work through a tragedy, and it has brought glory to him.

It is said that someone who has a brain injury will never be the same again. I fought that and said that those people don't know my God. I understand now that our lives have changed forever, but they have changed for the better, and I would never want to go back to the way things were before. Life isn't perfect now; we still have daily struggles. However, now my eyes are open, and I can see how truly blessed we are.

> Lord, you are my God.
> You are my strength and my refuge,
> my help in time of need.
> When circumstances are too overwhelming,
> you surround me with your presence.
>
> My God, you are my shelter,

you shield me from the storms that break me down.
You are my ever-present help.

Tragedy surrounds me;
I am drowning in sorrow and uncertainty.
I feel alone and helpless,
yet, my Savior, you carry me;
You will never leave my side.

Understanding I have not,
but I trust in you oh, Lord;
I place my trust in you.
I praise you in the midst of my struggles.
You will restore my life;
God, you will make me whole again.

My lips shout of your great love;
I sing praises of your mercy and righteousness.
Only you, my God,
can deliver me.

Praise you oh, Lord!
You will deliver me!
I will speak of your mercy,
of your grace, of your healing hands
all the days of my life!

ENDNOTES

1 Tammy Maltby, The God Who Sees You (David C. Cook, 2012) 93.

2 Sharon Riddle, *Warring at the Window* (Olive Leaf Publications, 2004), 49.

3 Mike Slaughter, *Christmas Is Not Your Birthday* (Nashville: Abingdon Press, 2011), 29.

4 Charles Stanley, Handle With Prayer: Unwrap the Source of God's Strength for Living 2 (Colorado Springs: David C. Cook, 2011) 7.

5 Anne Graham Lotz, *Into the Word: 52 Life-Changing Bible Studies for Individuals and Groups* (Grand Rapids: Zondervan, 2010), 288.

6 Richard Selenic and Karla Dougherty, *Living with Brain Injury: A Guide for Families 2* (Birmingham: HealthSouth Press, 2001), 165–166.

7 Gary Thomas, *Sacred Marriage Gift Edition* (Grand Rapids: Zondervan, 2011), 21, 33.

8 Richard Selenic and Karla Dougherty, *Living with Brain Injury: A Guide for Families 2* (Birmingham: HealthSouth Press, 2001), 2.

9 K. P. Yohannan, *Revolution in World Missions* (Gospel for Asia Books, 2004), 69.

10 Barbara Janet Cooper, *The Other Survivor: Head Injury from a Wife's Perspective* (Barbara Janet Cooper, 2009), 51.

11 Brian Jones, *Second Guessing God: Hanging on When You Can't See His Plan* (Cincinnati: Standard Publishing, 2006), 52–53.

12 Barbara Johnson, Laughter is the Spice of Life "Suffering Is Like Baking a Cake" (Nashville: W Publishing Group, 2004), 180.

13 Charles Stanley, Handle With Prayer: Unwrap the Source of God's Strength for Living 2 (Colorado Springs: David C. Cook, 2011), 7.

14 K.P. Yohannan, *The Beauty of Christ Through Brokenness* (Gospel for Asia Books, 2004), 39.

15 Brian Jones, *Second Guessing God: Hanging on When You Can't See His Plan* (Cincinnati: Standard Publishing, 2006), 37.

16 Kyle Idleman, *Not a Fan: Becoming a Completely Committed Follower of Jesus* (Zondervan, 2011), 136–137.

17 Ibid., 158.

BIBLIOGRAPHY

Cooper, Barbara Janet. *The Other Survivor: Head Injury from a Wife's Perspective.* Barbara Janet Cooper, 2009.

Idleman, Kyle. *Not a Fan: Becoming a Completely Committed Follower of Jesus.* Zondervan, 2011.

Johnson, Barbara. "Suffering is Like Baking a Cake." In *Laughter is the Spice of Life.* W Publishing Group, 2004.

Jones, Brian. *Second Guessing God: Hanging on When You Can't See His Plan.* Cincinnati: Standard Publishing, 2006.

Lotz, Anne Graham. *Into the Word: 52 Life-Changing Bible Studies for Individuals and Groups.* Zondervan, 2010.

Maltby, Tammy. *The God Who Sees You.* Colorado Springs: David C. Cook, 2012.

Riddle, Sharon. *Waiting at the Window.* Olive Leaf Publications, 2004.

Sclenic, Richard and Karla Dougherty. *Living with Brain Injury: A Guide for Families 2.* Birmingham: HealthSouth Press, 2001.

Slaughter, Mike. *Christmas Is Not Your Birthday.* Nashville: Abingdon Press, 2011.

Stanley, Charles. Handle With Prayer: Unwrap the Source of God's Strength for Living, 2. Colorado Springs: David C. Cook, 2011.

Thomas, Gary. *Sacred Marriage Gift Edition.* Grand Rapids: Zondervan, 2011.

Woodruff, Bob and Lee Woodruff. *In an Instant: A Family's Journey of Love and Healing.* New York: Random House Trade Paperbacks, 2008.

Yohannan, K. P. *The Beauty of Christ through Brokenness.* Gospel for Asia Books, 2004.